Mastering Your Fertility

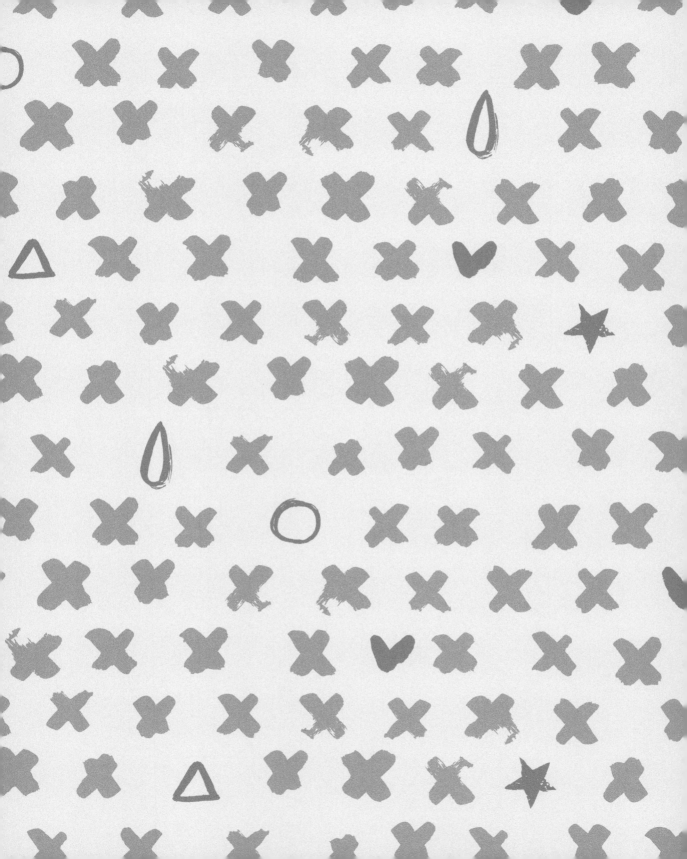

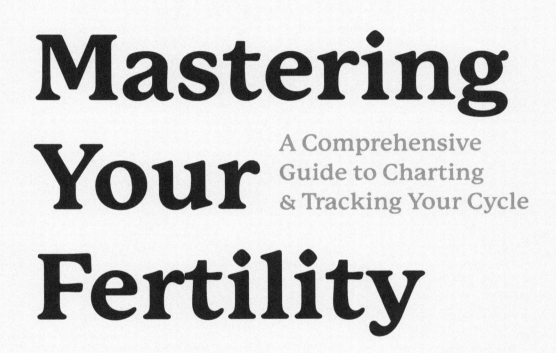

Mastering Your Fertility

A Comprehensive Guide to Charting & Tracking Your Cycle

Keeley McNamara, CNM

ROCKRIDGE
PRESS

Interior and Cover Designer: Emma Hall
Art Producer: Hillary Frileck
Editor: Claire Yee
Production Manager: Riley Hoffman
Production Editor: Melissa Edeburn

Illustration ©Shutterstock/Tsuyna, pages 23, 97, 98, and 99; ©Shutterstock/peart, page 9

Author photo courtesy of ©Sara Moe.

ISBN: Print 978-1-64152-784-2 | eBook 978-1-64152-785-9

R0

This book is dedicated to Evin, Winter, and Willa,
and to my family, friends, and midwife family.
Thank you for teaching, supporting,
believing in, and loving me so completely.

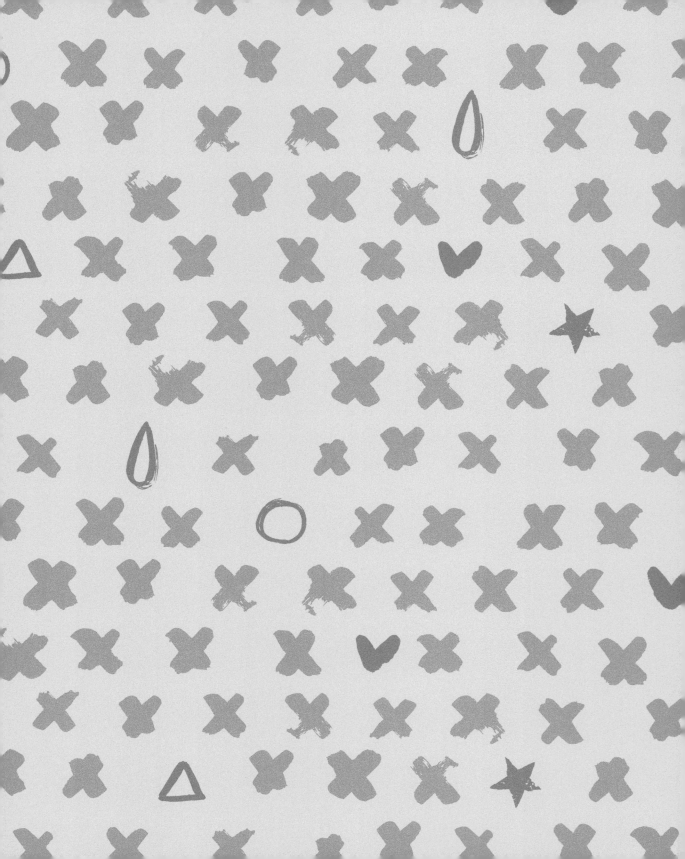

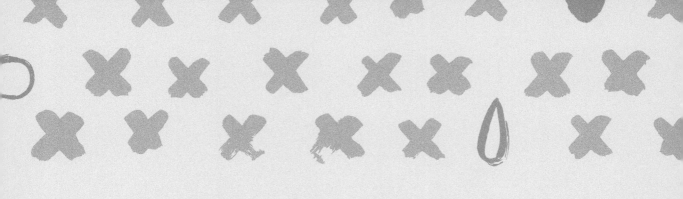

INTRODUCTION ix

1. **Listen to Your Body Talk** 1

2. **It Begins with a Period** 13

3. **Your Cycle Has Phases, Just Like the Moon** 19

4. **Let's Chart!** 27

5. **Decoding Your Cycle** 87

6. **Why Doesn't My Chart Look Like That?** 95

CONCLUSION 117

RESOURCES 118

REFERENCES 120

INDEX 124

Introduction

Hi, I'm Keeley. I started out my career as a sexual health educator. I later became a registered nurse and finally a certified nurse midwife. I have spent my professional life teaching women how to and how not to conceive, supporting them from menarche through menopause.

Whether I'm providing preconception counseling to a woman with a PhD or menopause counseling to a woman with 20 grandkids, I find that many of us are misinformed about how our bodies work. We know the basics about our menstrual cycle, like why and how often we menstruate, but other details are fuzzy. Some of us learn bits and pieces from our moms or aunties. Others of us have picked up information from books or rudimentary sex education courses. Many of us get misinformation from well-meaning friends (it's not like they went to some secret menstrual cycle and fertility class that you missed). Most of us just wing it and assume everything is working fine or that everything is broken until proven otherwise.

If you're reading this book, chances are that you're thinking about getting pregnant. Or you would very much like to not get pregnant. Or you're tired of having to bleach your sheets every month and want to understand your crazy, unpredictable periods. These are all amazing reasons to learn about your cycle by way of a fertility awareness method (and certainly better than learning how to get bloodstains out of cotton percale). But really, the most important reason is that understanding your menstrual cycle can help you take control of your overall health and fertility. No one knows your body better than you; not me, not your partner, not your health care provider. You simply need the tools to understand what your cycle is trying to tell you so that you can feel empowered.

For ease of use, this book is color coded! The colors directly correlate with one of the four phases of the menstrual cycle. Anything related to the menstruation phase is in BURGUNDY, anything related to the follicular phase is in PINK, anything related to ovulation is in PURPLE, and anything related to the luteal phase is in BLUE.

Chapter 1

Listen to Your Body Talk

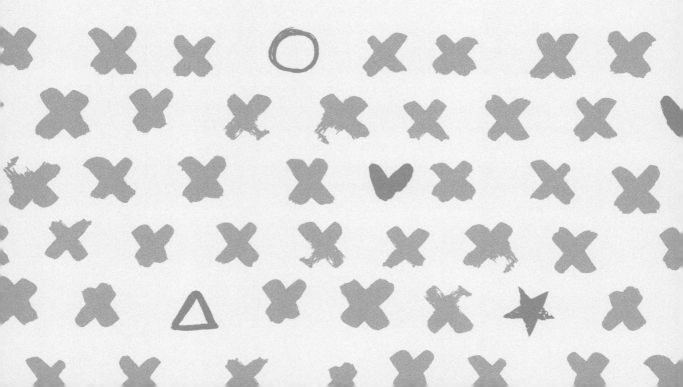

Your menstrual cycle is more than just your period. In fact, the days that you bleed are likely the least important days of your cycle even though they're probably the only ones you've ever given any attention (they're needy like that). The business of your menstrual cycle happens in between periods, in the hormone surges, in the consistency of cervical fluid and the position of your cervix, in your sharp shooting pain or your cramps and bloating, and in your almost imperceptible rise in body temperature. The fertility awareness method helps you interpret all the clues your body is giving you so that you can determine what your menstrual cycle is trying to tell you. This book will give you the tools you need to fully understand what your menstrual cycle reveals about your overall health. It explains how to chart and interpret your cycle.

REAL TALK

These are actual statements that I have heard from women in my personal and professional life and my initial reaction to them:

"My period is irregular. It comes at a different time every month."
  Does it come a different *day* in your cycle every month or a different *date* on the calendar every month?

"I get my period every month. I'm sure I will have no problem getting pregnant."
  But how do you know you're not having anovulatory cycles?

"Wait, what's an anovulatory cycle?"
  Anovulatory cycles happen when your body does not ovulate.

"My periods have never been an issue. I get one every three to four months and never have any PMS symptoms."
  This one's not just irregular but could also be dangerous.

"I have been having sex for over 10 years and have never gotten pregnant so I'm sure I'm infertile."
  That's luck, my friend. Pure luck. Or possibly not, but we can't tell from your lack of unplanned pregnancies alone.

  Let's decode all of this together!

What You Need to Know

You may be saying to yourself, "Who is she kidding? I don't have time for this. I'm mildly interested in the nitty-gritty information, but really, I'm just excited to unlock the secrets of my menstrual cycle." Great! Go through each chapter, find the "What You Need to Know" sections, and begin charting. It's like a Choose Your Own Adventure in fertility awareness.

How to begin:

1. Order a basal body thermometer (see the next page for details).

2. Continue to chapter 2.

3. Wait two interminably long days for your basal body thermometer to arrive.

4. While you're waiting, you might as well take this time to delve deeper. Read this chapter's "What You Really Should Know" section for more in-depth information. I mean, what else are you going to do with your two days? Sit around thinking about taking your temperature?

BASAL BODY THERMOMETER

You'll need to use a basal body thermometer to track your basal body temperature. A basal body thermometer is a special kind of thermometer that is accurate to every 0.1 degrees instead of every 0.2 degrees, like your typical thermometer. It is specifically designed to detect temperature changes that are associated with ovulation. Here are some key facts about basal body thermometers:

Key Facts about Basal Body Thermometers

- Basal body thermometers come in glass and digital versions.

- Glass thermometers are more accurate than digital ones, but you need to remember to shake them down at night and use them for at least five minutes before recording a reading.

- Vaginal and rectal temperatures are more accurate than oral. Any method can be used, just pick one and stick to it. If your oral temperature readings aren't making sense, try switching to vaginal or rectal for the next cycle.

- Take your temperature at the same time, in the same way, every day after at least three hours of uninterrupted sleep.

- Keep this book and your thermometer on your nightstand so you can take and record your temperature without moving around. It is important to take your temperature before doing anything else, including getting out of bed to fetch your thermometer from across the room.

- Change the alarm on your phone to read "Take My Temp" as a reminder.

- Don't forget to clean your thermometer every day—especially if you're taking vaginal or rectal temperatures. Just rinse the tip with warm water and a mild soap and leave it to air dry.

- Some digital thermometers indicate when the battery is low, but others do not. If it's taking a long time to register a temperature or your temperatures don't seem to be fluctuating, you should change the battery. It is best to change the battery during the menstruation phase of your cycle to avoid any inaccuracies in your chart.

What You Really Should Know

Basal body temperature, or waking temperature, is a valuable tool for you to learn about your hormones and cycle and to determine if you have ovulated. Before ovulation, your basal body temperature is suppressed by estrogen. After ovulation, progesterone takes over estrogen to prepare for a pregnancy. Progesterone is the hormone that makes us hot, which causes our temperature to rise. This temperature rise is basically your body turning into a human incubator for a possibly fertilized egg. Wait, did I say the rise happens *after* ovulation? Yes, I did. After ovulation. You are fertile in the five days prior to and the day of ovulation. That's why basal body temperature alone is not a good form of contraception. In fact, according to *Contraceptive Technology*, basal body temperature tracking alone has a failure rate of 13 percent to 20 percent among all users in clinical trials. The efficacy rate increases with the addition of other fertility indicators, such as cervical fluid or cervical position, but temperature alone should not be considered an effective method of contraception.

Over time, charting your temperature every day and every cycle will help you see the patterns of your hormones, but at first it's just going to look like a jumble of dots and line. I have included sample charts on pages 29 to 31 to help you figure out what your temperature is telling you about your body. The more you chart, the clearer the picture will become. Many women have told me that once they have it down, charting actually becomes a fun habit. Once you understand your natural fluctuation in hormones and how your medications, lifestyle, and diet can affect them, your body's changes throughout your cycle become much easier to predict.

The Four Menstrual Cycle Phases

Your menstrual cycle has four phases: the menstruation phase, the follicular phase, ovulation, and the luteal phase. Keep in mind that this book is color coded by phase on the charts and tabs whenever relevant. The menstruation phase lasts from the first to the last day of your period. It usually lasts between 3 and 8 days but averages 5 to 6 days for most women. The follicular phase starts on the first day of your period and lasts until you ovulate, which can be anywhere from 7 to 40 days. Yup, 40 days! Cycles can be weird. That's why it's important to understand them. Ovulation is the dividing line between the follicular and luteal phases of your menstrual cycle. Ovulation occurs when an egg is released from the ovary into the fallopian tube. The fourth phase of your cycle is the luteal phase, which lasts from the day of ovulation until the first day of your next period. The luteal phase is usually 12 to 16 days from the day of ovulation, with an average length of 14 days. The following figures show when the phases occur and how they overlap.

Diagram of Averages

MENSTRUATION	3 to 8 days (average 5 to 6 days)
FOLLICULAR PHASE	7 to 40 days (average 10 to 17 days)
OVULATION	dividing line between follicular & luteal phases
LUTEAL PHASE	12 to 16 days (average 14 days)

Menstrual Cycle

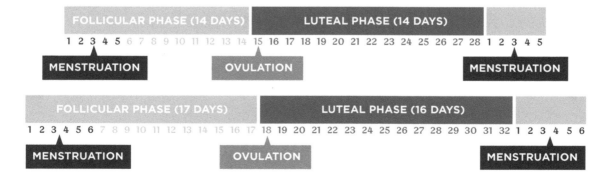

WHAT ABOUT MY CERVICAL FLUID?

According to *American Family Physician*, cervical fluid monitoring allows "users to identify the beginning and end of the fertile period by recognizing the cyclical changes in the amount or consistency of cervical secretions." There are multiple versions of this method, including the Creighton Model, the Billings Method, and the Two-Day Method, in which you ask yourself, "Did I note secretions today?" and "Did I note secretions yesterday?" The "yes secretions" days are your fertile days. Like your cervical fluid, the position of your cervix also changes throughout your cycle. Cervical position and cervical fluid alone should not be used to predict ovulation or prevent a pregnancy because they are open to interpretation and thus error. Although cervical fluid and position monitoring can be helpful when used in conjunction with basal body temperature (a method known as the sympto-thermal method), this book uses basal body temperature as the most prominent tool for better understanding your cycle and your body. It's easy to accurately collect and chart your temperature without too much room for error in interpretation.

Charting Your Cervical Fluid

The charts in this book provide some room for you to make note of cervical fluid. If you wish to better understand what your basal body temperature is telling you, charting your cervical fluid can be a good way to double-check your findings.

Sometimes when you take off your underwear, it is mysteriously wet. The wetness comes from normal cervical fluid. Almost every day, a woman will come to my office and ask me to fix her vaginal discharge. Most of the time, I have the same answer: Some vaginal discharge is totally normal. Having more or less throughout your cycle is also totally normal.

During ovulation, your body produces cervical fluid that mimics semen to help sperm make their way to your egg. In a man's body, sperm live and travel in semen, and without a substance like semen, sperm cannot move or survive. Without increased cervical fluid, sperm won't live long enough to make it to an egg for fertilization. It can be helpful to chart the consistency of your cervical fluid to help you pinpoint the time of ovulation. Cervical fluid is controlled by estrogen, so it changes throughout your menstrual cycle with your changing estrogen levels.

CONTINUED

You will have the least amount of cervical fluid immediately following menstruation. You may notice that your cervix is dry during this time. As the follicular phase progresses, your cervical fluid will become clear, cloudy, or yellow and will start to feel sticky, like rubber cement or white paste.

As ovulation nears, your cervical fluid will increase and become creamier, like lotion. The most fertile cervical fluid occurs during ovulation. It looks and feels like raw egg whites. It is extremely slippery and stretchy. It is usually clear, but it can also be tinged yellow or pink.

After ovulation, the amount of cervical fluid quickly decreases, and the texture becomes thicker due to the rapid drop in estrogen and rise in progesterone. The following figures show how your cervical fluid changes throughout your cycle.

To check your cervical fluid, look at the discharge on your underwear, wipe the opening of your vagina with toilet paper before you pee, or insert a clean finger into your vagina and try to find your cervix (hint: it's as far back as you can go at the end of your vagina). Rub and pull your cervical fluid between your thumb and index finger to check for slipperiness, stretchiness, and color before marking it on your chart.

Cervical Fluid and Your Cycle

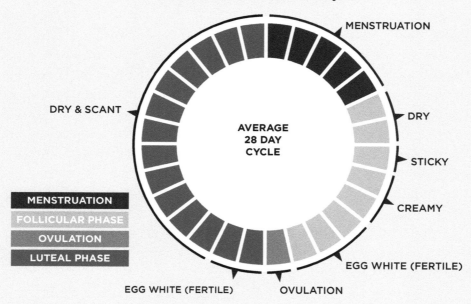

MENSTRUATION

DRY & SCANT

DRY

STICKY

AVERAGE
28 DAY
CYCLE

CREAMY

MENSTRUATION
FOLLICULAR PHASE
OVULATION
LUTEAL PHASE

EGG WHITE (FERTILE)

EGG WHITE (FERTILE)

OVULATION

Four Types of Cervical Fluid

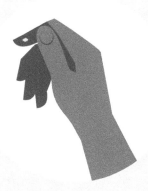

NOT OVULATING
dry, sticky

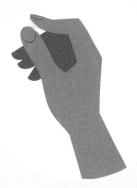

CLOSE TO OVULATION
wet, watery

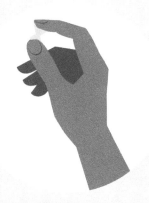

EVEN CLOSER TO OVULATION
creamy

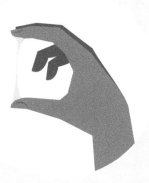

OVULATION
very wet, stretchy, egg white texture

Questions You'll End Up Asking

Q: Why is my cycle longer or shorter than 28 days, and why does it change from cycle to cycle?

A: The idea that your cycle should restart every 28 days and that you should ovulate on day 14 of that cycle is a myth. In reality, the average cycle ranges from 24 to 36 days and can differ from woman to woman—and, in each woman, from cycle to cycle. Ovulation usually occurs 12 to 16 days before your next period. By charting your cycle, you will learn whether and why you have an irregularly long or short cycle. The charts in this book can be tailored to cycles between 28 and 35 days long, so longer-than-average cycles won't be an issue.

Q: I've charted for one whole cycle. How much longer do I have to keep charting?

A: Ideally, you should chart at least three cycles before drawing any conclusions, especially if you typically have irregular periods or your charts differ from cycle to cycle. The goal is to begin detecting the patterns in your cycle.

Q: I'm not seeing any patterns in my charts.

A: Some factors can make charting inaccurate. According to the Mayo Clinic, illness, stress, travel, shift work, interrupted sleep or oversleeping, sedatives, alcohol, and time zone differences can all change your basal body temperature. Don't panic. You can still chart, just make a note of any irregularities to your normal routine on your chart so that you can explain the outlying temperatures. If you notice that the same activities are causing a disruption to your charting cycle after cycle, you may want to try eliminating them for a few cycles.

If your chart indicates that something may be abnormal, look at the list of possible next steps and questions on pages 35 and 36 to help guide you to the appropriate medical professional.

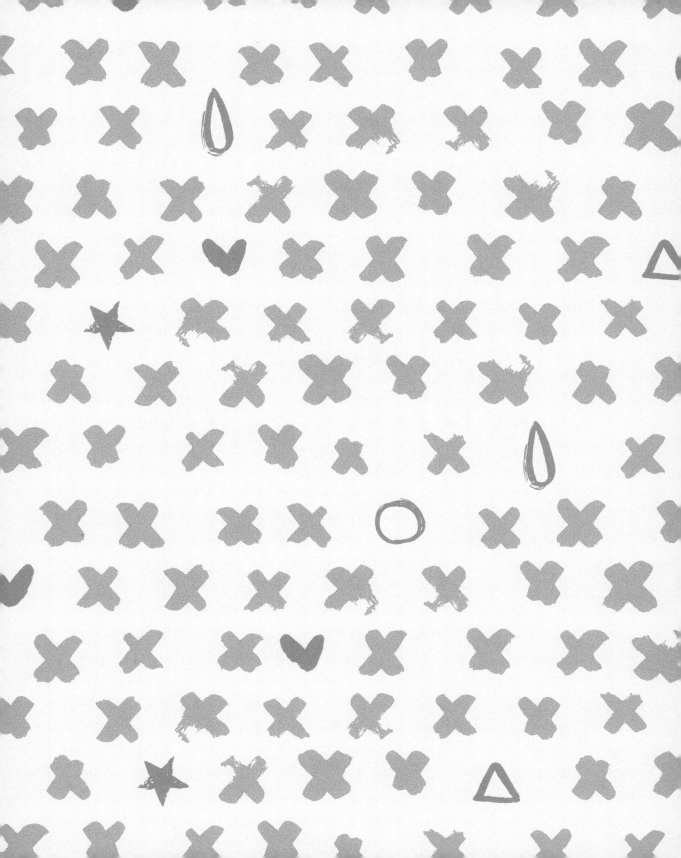

Chapter 2

It Begins
with a Period

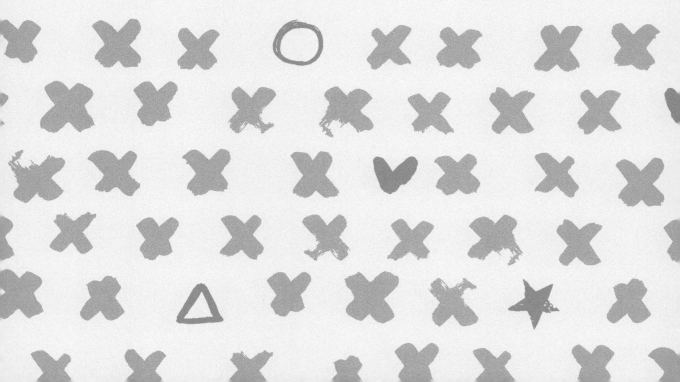

Welcome to the world of charting, and congratulations on making the commitment to learn what your body has been trying to tell you! You can use the fertility awareness method to prevent a pregnancy, to help you get pregnant, or to understand your cycle. So versatile!

Birth control failure rates vary from method to method, and the fertility awareness method is no different. According to the Centers for Disease Control and Prevention (CDC), with perfect use, the fertility awareness method failure rate can be as low as 2 percent. Too bad most of us aren't perfect. So yes, although you can technically use basal body temperature as a form of birth control, it typically is only 80 percent to 87 percent effective. Most women are not comfortable relying on a method with such a high failure rate.

That said, the fertility awareness method is a wonderful method to use if you are trying to get pregnant, to understand your cycle, or to use in conjunction with another method of birth control. Innumerable communities in the digital world can support you on your journey to understanding your cycle through basal body temperature charting. The Fertility Awareness Center and *Taking Charge of Your Fertility* have been around in support group and book form since the 1980s and now have an online presence as well. There is a list of resources at the end of this book if you are looking for additional information or communities.

What You Need to Know

Charting is taking your temperature every morning, recording that temperature in charts, like the ones provided in this book, and looking for the patterns that emerge over time. Easy, right? Kind of. As you can imagine, there is more nuance than just those three easy steps, but if you really want to boil it down, that's all there is to it. Take your temperature at the same time, in the same way, every day after at least three hours of uninterrupted sleep.

I've said this before, but it's super important, so I'm going to say it again: You need to take your temperature before you do anything else, including talking, eating, drinking, kissing, checking your phone, or moving around in bed. This really is the most important part of taking your temperature. I recommend that you set a repeating alarm labeled "Take My Temperature" in your phone. Your phone can help you remember even if your brain forgets! Keep this book and your thermometer on your nightstand. When your alarm goes off, remember why you set it in the first place, and immediately take your basal body temperature. Record it and then move on to all the kissing, eating in bed, and talking that your heart desires.

The temperatures you collect, record, and interpret will eventually reveal information about the length of the different phases of your cycle. From this information, you can determine critical aspects of your health, if and when you ovulate, if you might be pregnant, and when you can expect your next period.

Your menstrual cycle starts on the first day of your period, not the last. This is an incredibly important but often misunderstood fact about a woman's cycle. If you do not start charting on day one of your cycle, the chart will be invalid. If you have the kind of period where you spot or stain for a day or two prior to your first real day of bleeding, you may be tempted to count the first drop of blood as day one. I know you've been waiting anxiously to start charting, but hold on just a day or two more. Those spotty days are important, but day one of your cycle is the first day of red blood as opposed to brown or pink staining. There is a section in our charts where you can chart the flow of your period. If you feel that you know all you need to know to get started, you can move straight to the chart at this point. If you want to learn more before you start charting, move to the "What You Really Should Know" section of this chapter.

HOW CAN I RELATE?

Meet Elizabeth. Elizabeth spent the majority of her 20s happily on birth control pills, but after she had kids in her 30s, she realized her period was not as regular as she had thought. She decided that she wanted to try to understand her cycle rather than suppress it.

When I was on the pill, my period came every 28 days, like clockwork. It wasn't until after I stopped them that I realized it wasn't my cycle at all but the pills that were on time. At first I was overwhelmed by the idea of basal body temperature charting. I wasn't sure I would even be able to remember to take my temperature every morning, let alone record and understand it. I'm a working mom of two, so I don't have a lot of time to spare and was worried that I would spend all this time taking and recording my temperature, and it would be a waste of my time. I decided to commit to at least trying, and after a few weeks, taking and tracking my temperature became part of my routine. My best advice is to just keep charting. At first it does look like a crazy game of connect the dots, but eventually those dots and lines come into focus and start making sense.

What You Really Should Know

Code Red. Shark Week. On the rag. Defrosting the steak (Spain). Blood festival (Japan). There are over 5,000 slang terms for *period* around the world, but I've never heard any pithy way to say ovulation, cervical fluid, luteal phase, or mittelschmerz (ovulation pain). No one even talks about, let alone jokes about, the other phases of your menstrual cycle because the other phases are not messy or dangerous. The other phases don't insinuate that sex has or has not occurred. We don't hear or learn about cervical fluid because there is nothing sexy or precarious about cervical fluid.

We get our information about our bodies from many different sources, many of which are not particularly positive or correct. In school, it was in a class where the boys were sent out of the room and your teacher awkwardly dunked a tampon into a cup of water so you could see how much blood it would hold. On television, periods are portrayed in an amusing and mildly terrifying scene where some poor girl's first period comes on the day of the big beach party in her new white bathing suit. In my experience, however, most of us learned the majority of what we know from our friends. From talking about pads and tampons with our bunkmates in camp to discussing post-baby periods and handling perimenopausal hemorrhaging with our mom friends, every group of women I know in every stage of their lives eventually starts sharing experiences about their periods.

The Science of Your Cycle

I'm going to get technical here for those of you who want to understand the science of your cycle. To help you visualize what's happening with your body, refer back to the figure on page 6 to see the overlaps, variations, and averages of each phase. Don't worry if this all seems like a foreign language—you don't have to understand it to understand charting.

Your menstrual cycle is not just your period. Your menstrual cycle is an intricate but perfectly designed call and response. If one part is delayed or suppressed, another part is directly affected and will adjust accordingly. Your menstrual cycle starts on the first day of your period when your estrogen level is low. Your brain then releases follicle stimulating hormones (FSH) that trigger follicles in the ovaries to mature. As the follicles mature, they release more and more estrogen. These high levels of estrogen tell your brain that there is a mature egg ready, and luteinizing hormones (LH) are then released.

It can take anywhere from 8 days to 40 days for estrogen levels to get high enough to trigger the LH surge, which, in turn, triggers ovulation and tells one of your ovaries to release an egg. The period of time from ovulation through the start of your next period is known as the luteal phase. The mature egg is released about 24 to 36 hours after the LH surge and travels down the fallopian tube, while the corpus luteum (the follicle from which the egg was released) produces progesterone. Remember our friend progesterone, the hormone that causes our basal body temperature to rise? This is progesterone's moment to shine. The corpus luteum produces progesterone for 12 to 16 days or, if a pregnancy occurs, until the placenta takes over at around eight weeks. Heat-producing progesterone is only released once ovulation has occurred, which is why the rise in basal body temperature in your chart indicates that ovulation has already occurred.

There are apps that can help you track your period, your basal body temperature, your cervical fluid, or some combination of all three. These apps use algorithms designed to match your input to the most common cycle patterns programmed into it. Though they are convenient, many women prefer written charting to truly understand the details of why their cycle is the way it is rather than just getting the overview. You may also choose to use both at once as a way to double-check your written charts.

Knowing and understanding the length of your follicular phase, your day of ovulation, the length of your luteal phase, and the length and characteristics of your menstruation phase can tell you about hormone imbalances; the effect stress, medications, and nutrition have on your body; and certain medical conditions and endocrine disorders. In chapter 6, I go into much more detail and provide samples of what your charts might look like due to different hormone imbalances, lifestyle choices, and medical conditions.

Chapter 3

Your Cycle Has Phases, Just Like the Moon

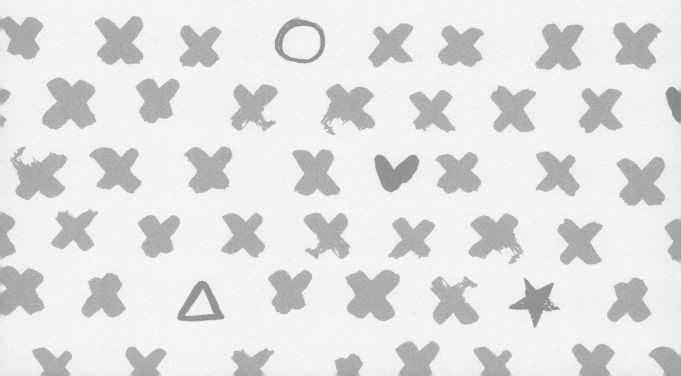

Your menstrual cycle has four phases. The moon has four phases. Your menstrual cycle lasts about 29.5 days. The moon cycle lasts about 29.5 days. The full moon is about 15 days before the new moon. Most women ovulate about 15 days before their next period. The moon is made out of cheese. Your menstrual cycle . . . I'm just kidding.

Since the beginning of time, women have linked their menstrual cycles to the lunar cycle, and many cultures believe that the menstrual cycle is directly affected by the moon cycle. Even the words *menstruation* and *menses* come from the Latin and Greek words meaning month (*mensis*) and moon (*mene*). According to some cultures, if you menstruate in a new moon and ovulate in a full moon, your body is on the White Moon Cycle. Your ovulation takes place during the time of the full moon when the world is most fertile. Plants grow better, the tides are higher, and ovaries release eggs with the full moon. Legend has it that women on this cycle pattern mother, nurture, and raise children. Alternatively, if you menstruate with a full moon, it's called a Red Moon Cycle. It is said that these women are the healers who spill their blood into the rebirth of the world. They are the witches, artists, healers, and midwives.

Menstrual Moon Cycle

MENSTRUATION
new moon

FOLLICULAR
waxing moon

LUTEAL
waning moon

OVULATION
full moon

Although this is all fun to think about, the reality is that there is no scientific evidence of syncing menstrual and lunar cycles. Sure, some women will ovulate with the full moon or the new moon, but evidence shows that women are just as likely to ovulate at any other time in the lunar cycle. Charting using the fertility awareness method may be less whimsical than charting lunar cycles, but it is a far more reliable way of figuring out when you ovulate.

What You Need to Know

"Do I have a healthy cycle, and can I get pregnant?"

That's what we aim to find out. Statistically speaking, probably. Ninety-five percent of all cycles are between 15 and 45 days long, and 90 percent of women will be able to get pregnant within one year of trying to conceive. Those are pretty good odds, so why do you need this book? Because not everyone wants to conceive. And not everyone wants to wait a year to get pregnant. And most importantly, because you want to understand your body and why it does what it does.

Let's review the four phases of the menstrual cycle. Refer back to the figure on page 6 when reviewing the following list for a diagram of the average lengths of phases in a menstrual cycle. If you ever want to learn more specifically about one phase over another, this book is color coded by phase on the charts and tabs.

Menstruation

The menstruation phase starts on the first day of your period and ends on the last day of your period. This phase varies cycle to cycle and woman to woman, but for most women it lasts between three and eight days and averages between five and six days. Spotting before a period is usually brown or rust-colored, whereas real menstrual bleeding can range from light pink to bright red. The average woman loses two teaspoons of blood over the course of her menstruation phase.

Follicular

The follicular phase starts on the first day of your period, overlaps the menstruation phase, and ends on the day you ovulate. During the follicular phase, estrogen levels rise as a dominant follicle develops in the ovary. The rise in estrogen is what causes ovulation to occur. This is the phase that varies the most between cycles and can last anywhere from 8 to 40 days, averaging 10 to 17 days.

Ovulation

The ovulation phase is the day of ovulation. The rising estrogen levels that occur during the follicular phase finally reach the level of your body's estrogen threshold and cause a surge of luteinizing hormone (LH). The follicle releases a mature egg from the ovary, usually within 24 to 36 hours of the LH surge, when the egg is swept into the fallopian tube and begins its trip to the uterus.

Luteal

The luteal phase starts on the day of ovulation and ends the day before your next period starts. After releasing the egg, the follicle left behind becomes a corpus luteum, which produces progesterone. The corpus luteum only lives and produces progesterone for 12 to 16 days. The decline in progesterone is what triggers your next period to start. The luteal phase has much less variation than the follicular phase, as it lasts only as long as the corpus luteum lasts.

A woman can only get pregnant in the five days before ovulation and the day of ovulation. However, being knowledgeable of all phases through the fertility awareness method is equally important to understanding your period, your ability to conceive, your body, and your health.

Okay, that's it! You understand the phases of your cycle and the color coding of this book. If you're ready to get going, move on to chapter 4 and get charting.

What You Really Should Know

Though it is true that you can only get pregnant around the time of ovulation, fertility actually has to do with phases other than ovulation. Some women ovulate but have a short luteal phase, otherwise known as a luteal phase defect. A short luteal phase lasts less than 10 days and occurs when a woman's body does not produce enough progesterone. When this happens, the uterine or endometrial lining doesn't get thick enough for a pregnancy to implant. For these women, the issue is not ovulation, but the short time between ovulation and menstruation. If this interval is too short, the pregnancy simply does not have time to stick. These early pregnancy losses are called chemical pregnancies and account for 50 percent to 70 percent of all miscarriages. A chemical pregnancy is a miscarriage that occurs before the fifth week of pregnancy, when it is too early for the pregnancy to be seen on ultrasound but not to be detected by blood work. Most of these chemical pregnancies end about one week after a woman's menstruation was due, so unless you are trying for a pregnancy and testing early, you may not even realize a pregnancy and miscarriage have occurred—you may just think your period was a little later and a little heavier than normal that cycle.

The Uterine Lining

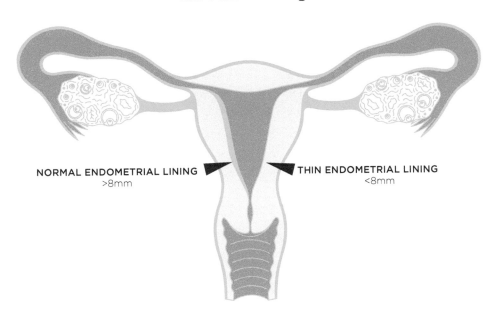

NORMAL ENDOMETRIAL LINING
>8mm

THIN ENDOMETRIAL LINING
<8mm

Some women, however, ovulate rarely or not at all. This is called an anovulatory cycle. Anovulatory cycles are very normal in the years following your first period and in the years leading up to menopause. It is also very common and normal for women to have one or two anovulatory cycles per year. An anovulatory cycle can be sporadic (when a woman skips ovulation once in a while) or can be chronic (when a woman has less than eight menstrual cycles per year). If your cycle is shorter than 21 days or longer than 36 days, it could be a sign of an anovulatory cycle. Your cycles may also be anovulatory if the length varies drastically from cycle to cycle. When anovulatory cycles occur, the lining of your uterus eventually sheds, either as light spotting or heavy bleeding, called breakthrough bleeding. Anovulatory cycles can be caused by hormonal imbalances, being underweight or obese, stress, or some medications, including NSAIDs. It is also common to have a few anovulatory cycles after you stop hormonal birth control.

Once you start charting, you'll be able to tell how many menstrual cycles you have per year and if you have an average or shorter-than-average luteal phase as well as any other abnormalities in your cycle. You are unlikely to have a long luteal phase unless you become pregnant that cycle. Every woman should have her period at least once every three months to avoid a thickened endometrial lining, which can be dangerous if left untreated. If you notice that you are going longer than three months without a period, you should go to your health care provider. You may need testing done to see if you have a condition that can cause chronic anovulation such as PCOS, endometriosis, thyroid disease, or a sexually transmitted infection. You may need medication to induce a period or to fix a hormonal imbalance so your period can come on its own. You may be asked to lose or gain weight or make changes to your lifestyle to reduce excessive stress. Bring your charts with you to your appointment. They will help give your provider a clearer picture of what is happening with your cycle and your body.

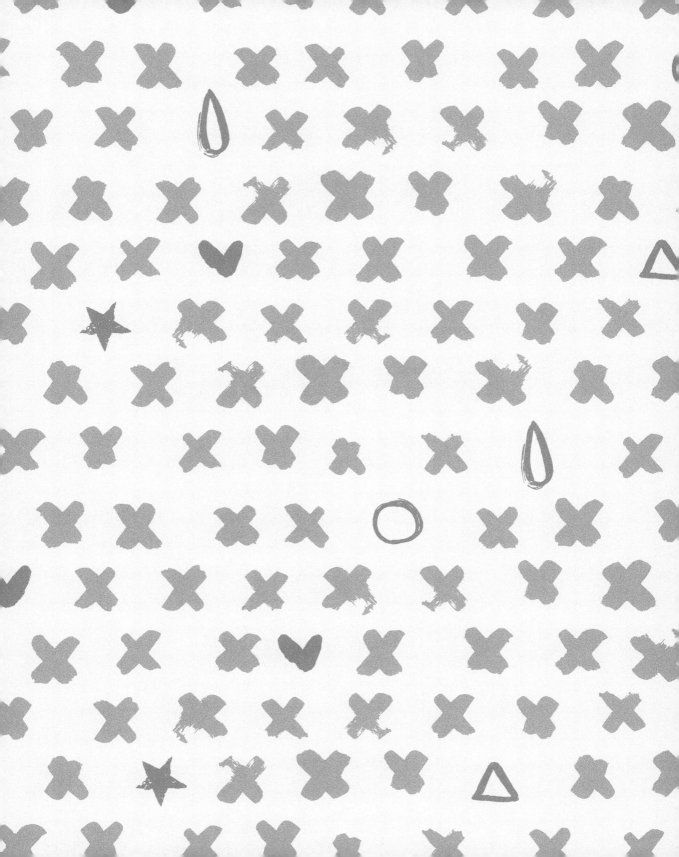

Chapter 4

Let's Chart!

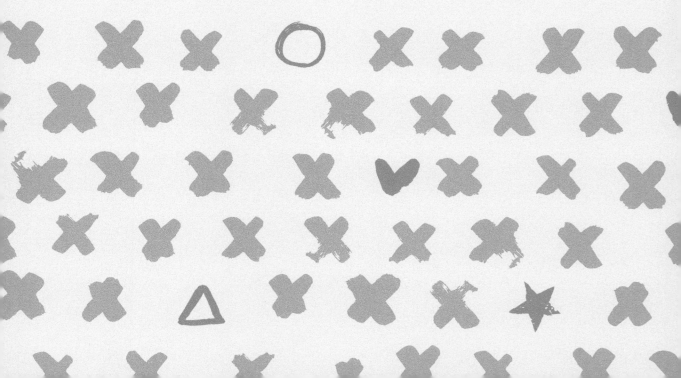

Reader, meet your new friend: your fertility awareness method chart. It is designed to be easier for you to use than the one-size-fits-all charts you find on the Internet or in apps. You and your chart might as well get to know each other because you'll be spending every morning together from here on out.

This chart is color coded to match up with the phases of your cycle, gradually changing as the next phase gets closer. As long as you are charting your phase within the color associated with that phase, your cycle is probably normal. If something in your chart is confusing, turn to the sections of this book that correlate to the color of the phase you're trying to figure out, and read up! The answers are all at your fingertips.

Let's start at the top. Your chart starts with cycle day one; underneath that you should write the date, day of the week, and time you took your temperature. There are places to mark if you had sex that day and to describe your cervical fluid and menstrual flow. Next, you will find your basal body temperature chart for every 0.1 degrees. There is also room to make notes about anything unusual. This is where you may want to note if you woke up earlier or later than normal or if you drank alcohol the night before, which could raise your waking temperature. This way, if there are any irregularities in your cycle, you can see what might be affecting it. If you find that you need more room, feel free to jot down detailed notes in a journal.

See the keys on the next page for cervical fluid and menstrual flow charting abbreviations.

Cervical Fluid Key

N	none (dry, no cervical fluid present)
S	sticky (pasty, sticky like rubber cement, usually white or yellow; sits on top of underwear)
C	creamy (like lotion, milky, smooth, usually white or yellow; sits on top of underwear)
E	egg white and/or slippery (slippery, stretches an inch or more between thumb and index finger, clear, streaked, or opaque; wet, may sit on top of or soak into underwear)

Menstrual Flow Key

S	spotting (brown or rust-colored discharge)
L	light (pink or red, light flow)
M	medium (red, moderate flow, needing to change pads/tampons/menstrual cups as recommended)
H	heavy (red, needing to change pads/tampons/menstrual cups more frequently than recommended, possibly with blood clots)

SAMPLE BASAL BODY TEMPERATURE CHARTS

Here are three examples of what charts for a woman with a healthy cycle may look like.

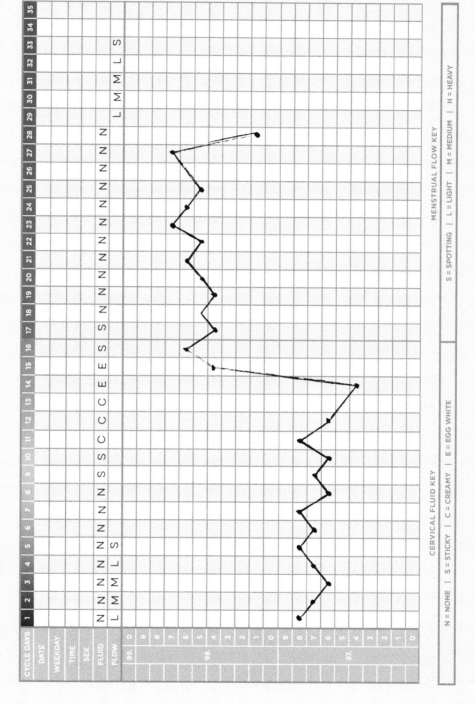

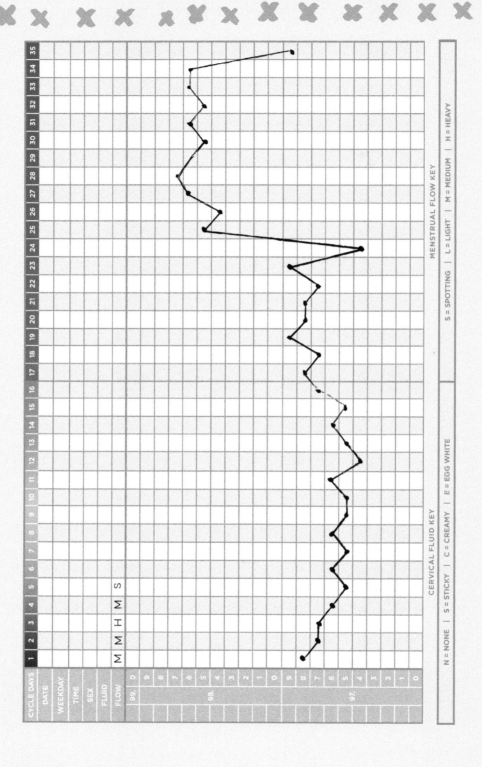

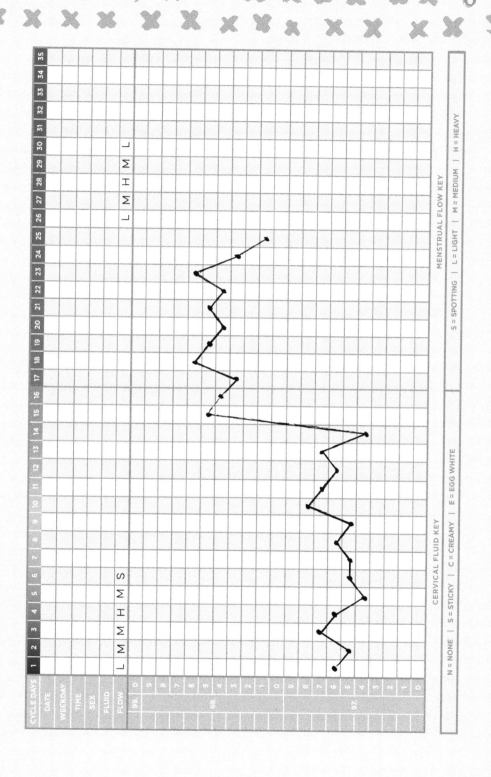

What You Need to Know

The charts in this book are different from other charts because they are the most awesome charts that ever charted. Too much? Fine. But they are color coded according to cycle phase, which makes them much easier to use. These color codes match pertinent reference tabs and diagrams throughout the book. Notice the ombre color shift between phases? That ombre area shows you the normal range for that phase. This takes some of the guesswork out of trying to interpret your chart. Simply identify which color corresponds to the section of your chart about which you want to learn more and flip to those color-coded tabs. Maybe your period comes like clockwork every month, but you have a longer follicular phase than you realized. Flip around to the PINK tabs and learn all there is to know about your long follicular phase and what it could be telling you about your overall health.

You want to pay close attention to each phase of your cycle and ask yourself questions like these:

- Does my menstruation phase start or end with spotting?

- Is my period particularly heavy with clots? Does it last longer than seven days?

- Is my follicular phase a typical 14 days, or is it much longer or shorter?

- Do I notice egg white cervical fluid for more of my cycle than just during ovulation?

- Are my periods much lighter or shorter than average?

You'll probably see the most variation on the length of your follicular phase, as stress or illness can delay ovulation. Maybe you've realized that your regular 28-day cycle is actually a 20-day follicular phase followed by an 8-day luteal phase, and what you thought was a normal cycle is actually anything but. Whatever you discover, chapter 6 and the Resources section at the end of this book on page 118 will help you figure out what steps to take next.

If you skipped straight ahead to charting and are now feeling a bit confused by your charts, don't worry. It's totally normal to feel confused at first. You can always go back to the "What You Really Should Know" section in chapter 3 on page 23 for a deeper look into the four menstrual cycal phases. Learning more about the phases of your menstrual cycle can help you understand what your chart reveals about your body and overall health.

HOW CAN I RELATE?

Meet Jen. Jen got her period every month for four to six days like clockwork. Some cycles, she would have a little brown spotting at the beginning of her period, but she never really paid attention to it. Jen assumed she would have no trouble getting pregnant since her periods were regular, but after six months of trying, she had not conceived.

My doctor wouldn't start infertility testing until I had been trying for at least one year, but I felt like I had to do something. I did a little research and decided to try the fertility awareness method. When I started, I didn't even know that there were phases of my menstrual cycle. I honestly thought all that mattered was that my period was coming. I took my temperature every morning and checked and recorded my cervical fluid. I soon realized that I was ovulating every month like I thought but that I have a short luteal cycle. To be clear, first I learned what a luteal phase was, then I found out mine was short. I brought my charts to my doctor, and he was able to do a simple blood test to confirm what I had discovered. I am now taking medication to help make my luteal phase longer and am feeling hopeful about a future pregnancy.

What You Really Should Know

There is a wide range in variation of phase lengths during your menstrual cycle. Most of these variations will land squarely in the realm of healthy even if they are different from the average length of the phase indicated. The follicular phase, for example, can be anywhere from 8 to 40 days long and still be normal. That being said, the average is 10 to 17 days, and it usually shortens as you near menopause. Though a very short or long follicular phase can be a normal part of the menstrual cycle, it can also be a sign of excess estrogen, which could be a sign of polycystic ovary syndrome (we'll talk about this in chapter 6). The luteal phase, on the other hand, should be between 12 and 16 days. Anything shorter than 10 days indicates low progesterone levels, which can lead to chemical pregnancies, or early miscarriages. Anything longer, and you may be pregnant.

You are now ready to start charting. Put your thermometer and this book next to your bed and wait for the first day of your next period to come. If you need to review anything, just refer to the color-coded tabs to find the phase of your menstrual cycle about which you want more information. You should chart for at least three cycles before looking for patterns in your charts. Once you've done that, read chapter 5 to decode your charts. You've got this! Get charting and start figuring out what your body is trying to tell you.

DON'T FREAK OUT!

Some common questions people ask when they start charting:

Q: Why aren't my days matching up with the example charts?
A: Everyone's chart will look different. There is no right or wrong chart. Just keep going so you can figure out what a normal chart looks like for you.

Q: Why isn't my temperature rising?
A: Read the first paragraph of the "What You Need and Really Should Know" section in chapter 5 on page 88 to make sure you know how to identify a temperature shift. If you aren't seeing a temperature rise on your chart, you may have had an anovulatory cycle. Everyone has an anovulatory cycle every once in a while, which can be caused by stress or illness. If you start to notice a pattern of anovulatory cycles, you may have a medical condition that is causing this. Notify your health care provider to evaluate possible anovulatory cycles.

Q: Did I ovulate too close to my period?
A: If your next period started less than 10 days after you ovulated, it could mean one of two things: Either you had a shorter luteal phase, meaning that your progesterone levels dropped before they should have, or your basal body temperature took a few days to show ovulation even though you have indeed already ovulated. If you feel like you ovulated, but your temperature rise isn't matching up, you may want to start charting your other signs of ovulation, such as cervical fluid, as a way to pinpoint more exactly when your ovulation is occurring.

Q: Help! I forgot to take my temperature before I got up!
A: It's okay if you forget one day, just be extra careful to remember the next day. Your chart may be a little inaccurate that cycle, but it's not just about any single cycle, it's about noticing the patterns and changes over time. Mark on your chart that you forgot to take your temperature to remind yourself of this when you're reviewing your chart at a later time. The details of all those dots get a bit blurry over time, so it's important to note anything out of the ordinary.

Q: I bled a little for a day and then I stopped. Do I start a new chart?
A: Light spotting can be a sign of ovulation, implantation bleeding, low progesterone levels, a thyroid condition, uterine or cervical abnormality, medication side effects, or an infection. A true menstrual period only takes place after a 12- to 16-day temperature increase. Take note of the spotting on your chart, but do not count it as day one of your new cycle.

Basal Body Temperature Charts

Basal Body Temperature Chart

CYCLE DAYS		1	2	3	4	5	6	7	8	9	10	11	12	13	14	15	16
DATE																	
WEEKDAY																	
TIME																	
SEX																	
FLUID																	
FLOW																	
99.	0																
	9																
	8																
	7																
	6																
	5																
98.	4																
	3																
	2																
	1																
	0																
	9																
	8																
	7																
	6																
	5																
97.	4																
	3																
	2																
	1																
	0																
NOTES																	

CERVICAL FLUID KEY

N = NONE | S = STICKY | C = CREAMY | E = EGG WHITE

DATES:_____ to_____

17	18	19	20	21	22	23	24	25	26	27	28	29	30	31	32	33	34	35

MENSTRUAL FLOW KEY

S = SPOTTING | L = LIGHT | M = MEDIUM | H = HEAVY

Basal Body Temperature Chart

CYCLE DAYS		1	2	3	4	5	6	7	8	9	10	11	12	13	14	15	16
DATE																	
WEEKDAY																	
TIME																	
SEX																	
FLUID																	
FLOW																	
99.	0																
	9																
	8																
	7																
	6																
	5																
98.	4																
	3																
	2																
	1																
	0																
	9																
	8																
	7																
	6																
	5																
97.	4																
	3																
	2																
	1																
	0																
NOTES																	

CERVICAL FLUID KEY

N = NONE | S = STICKY | C = CREAMY | E = EGG WHITE

DATES:_____to_____

17	18	19	20	21	22	23	24	25	26	27	28	29	30	31	32	33	34	35

MENSTRUAL FLOW KEY

S = SPOTTING | L = LIGHT | M = MEDIUM | H = HEAVY

Basal Body Temperature Chart

CYCLE DAYS		1	2	3	4	5	6	7	8	9	10	11	12	13	14	15	16
DATE																	
WEEKDAY																	
TIME																	
SEX																	
FLUID																	
FLOW																	
99.	0																
	9																
	8																
	7																
	6																
	5																
98.	4																
	3																
	2																
	1																
	0																
	9																
	8																
	7																
	6																
	5																
97.	4																
	3																
	2																
	1																
	0																
NOTES																	

CERVICAL FLUID KEY

N = NONE | S = STICKY | C = CREAMY | E = EGG WHITE

DATES:_____ to_____

17	18	19	20	21	22	23	24	25	26	27	28	29	30	31	32	33	34	35

MENSTRUAL FLOW KEY

S = SPOTTING | L = LIGHT | M = MEDIUM | H = HEAVY

Basal Body Temperature Chart

CYCLE DAYS		1	2	3	4	5	6	7	8	9	10	11	12	13	14	15	16
DATE																	
WEEKDAY																	
TIME																	
SEX																	
FLUID																	
FLOW																	
99.	0																
	9																
	8																
	7																
	6																
	5																
98.	4																
	3																
	2																
	1																
	0																
	9																
	8																
	7																
	6																
	5																
97.	4																
	3																
	2																
	1																
	0																
NOTES																	

CERVICAL FLUID KEY

N = NONE | S = STICKY | C = CREAMY | E = EGG WHITE

DATES:_____to_____

17	18	19	20	21	22	23	24	25	26	27	28	29	30	31	32	33	34	35

MENSTRUAL FLOW KEY

S = SPOTTING | L = LIGHT | M = MEDIUM | H = HEAVY

Basal Body Temperature Chart

CYCLE DAYS		1	2	3	4	5	6	7	8	9	10	11	12	13	14	15	16
DATE																	
WEEKDAY																	
TIME																	
SEX																	
FLUID																	
FLOW																	
99.	0																
	9																
	8																
	7																
	6																
	5																
98.	4																
	3																
	2																
	1																
	0																
	9																
	8																
	7																
	6																
	5																
97.	4																
	3																
	2																
	1																
	0																
NOTES																	

CERVICAL FLUID KEY

N = NONE | S = STICKY | C = CREAMY | E = EGG WHITE

DATES:_____to_____

	17	18	19	20	21	22	23	24	25	26	27	28	29	30	31	32	33	34	35

MENSTRUAL FLOW KEY

S = SPOTTING | L = LIGHT | M = MEDIUM | H = HEAVY

Basal Body Temperature Chart

CYCLE DAYS		1	2	3	4	5	6	7	8	9	10	11	12	13	14	15	16
DATE																	
WEEKDAY																	
TIME																	
SEX																	
FLUID																	
FLOW																	
99.	0																
	9																
	8																
	7																
	6																
	5																
98.	4																
	3																
	2																
	1																
	0																
	9																
	8																
	7																
	6																
	5																
97.	4																
	3																
	2																
	1																
	0																
NOTES																	

CERVICAL FLUID KEY

N = NONE | S = STICKY | C = CREAMY | E = EGG WHITE

17	18	19	20	21	22	23	24	25	26	27	28	29	30	31	32	33	34	35

MENSTRUAL FLOW KEY

| S = SPOTTING | L = LIGHT | M = MEDIUM | H = HEAVY |

Basal Body Temperature Chart

CYCLE DAYS		1	2	3	4	5	6	7	8	9	10	11	12	13	14	15	16
DATE																	
WEEKDAY																	
TIME																	
SEX																	
FLUID																	
FLOW																	
99.	0																
	9																
	8																
	7																
	6																
	5																
98.	4																
	3																
	2																
	1																
	0																
	9																
	8																
	7																
	6																
	5																
97.	4																
	3																
	2																
	1																
	0																
NOTES																	

CERVICAL FLUID KEY

N = NONE | S = STICKY | C = CREAMY | E = EGG WHITE

DATES:_____to_____

	17	18	19	20	21	22	23	24	25	26	27	28	29	30	31	32	33	34	35

MENSTRUAL FLOW KEY

S = SPOTTING | L = LIGHT | M = MEDIUM | H = HEAVY

Basal Body Temperature Chart

CYCLE DAYS		1	2	3	4	5	6	7	8	9	10	11	12	13	14	15	16
DATE																	
WEEKDAY																	
TIME																	
SEX																	
FLUID																	
FLOW																	
99.	0																
	9																
	8																
	7																
	6																
	5																
98.	4																
	3																
	2																
	1																
	0																
	9																
	8																
	7																
	6																
	5																
97.	4																
	3																
	2																
	1																
	0																
NOTES																	

CERVICAL FLUID KEY

N = NONE | S = STICKY | C = CREAMY | E = EGG WHITE

17	18	19	20	21	22	23	24	25	26	27	28	29	30	31	32	33	34	35

MENSTRUAL FLOW KEY

S = SPOTTING | L = LIGHT | M = MEDIUM | H = HEAVY

Basal Body Temperature Chart

CYCLE DAYS		1	2	3	4	5	6	7	8	9	10	11	12	13	14	15	16
DATE																	
WEEKDAY																	
TIME																	
SEX																	
FLUID																	
FLOW																	
99.	0																
	9																
	8																
	7																
	6																
	5																
98.	4																
	3																
	2																
	1																
	0																
	9																
	8																
	7																
	6																
	5																
97.	4																
	3																
	2																
	1																
	0																
NOTES																	

CERVICAL FLUID KEY

N = NONE | S = STICKY | C = CREAMY | E = EGG WHITE

DATES:_____to_____

17	18	19	20	21	22	23	24	25	26	27	28	29	30	31	32	33	34	35

MENSTRUAL FLOW KEY

S = SPOTTING | L = LIGHT | M = MEDIUM | H = HEAVY

Basal Body Temperature Chart

CYCLE DAYS		1	2	3	4	5	6	7	8	9	10	11	12	13	14	15	16
DATE																	
WEEKDAY																	
TIME																	
SEX																	
FLUID																	
FLOW																	
99.	0																
	9																
	8																
	7																
	6																
	5																
98.	4																
	3																
	2																
	1																
	0																
	9																
	8																
	7																
	6																
	5																
97.	4																
	3																
	2																
	1																
	0																
NOTES																	

CERVICAL FLUID KEY

N = NONE | S = STICKY | C = CREAMY | E = EGG WHITE

17	18	19	20	21	22	23	24	25	26	27	28	29	30	31	32	33	34	35

MENSTRUAL FLOW KEY

S = SPOTTING | L = LIGHT | M = MEDIUM | H = HEAVY

Basal Body Temperature Chart

CYCLE DAYS	1	2	3	4	5	6	7	8	9	10	11	12	13	14	15	16
DATE																
WEEKDAY																
TIME																
SEX																
FLUID																
FLOW																
99. 0																
9																
8																
7																
6																
5																
98. 4																
3																
2																
1																
0																
9																
8																
7																
6																
5																
97. 4																
3																
2																
1																
0																
NOTES																

CERVICAL FLUID KEY

N = NONE | S = STICKY | C = CREAMY | E = EGG WHITE

DATES:_____ to_____

17	18	19	20	21	22	23	24	25	26	27	28	29	30	31	32	33	34	35

MENSTRUAL FLOW KEY

S = SPOTTING | L = LIGHT | M = MEDIUM | H = HEAVY

Basal Body Temperature Chart

CYCLE DAYS	1	2	3	4	5	6	7	8	9	10	11	12	13	14	15	16
DATE																
WEEKDAY																
TIME																
SEX																
FLUID																
FLOW																
99. 0																
9																
8																
7																
6																
5																
98. 4																
3																
2																
1																
0																
9																
8																
7																
6																
5																
97. 4																
3																
2																
1																
0																
NOTES																

CERVICAL FLUID KEY

N = NONE | S = STICKY | C = CREAMY | E = EGG WHITE

DATES:_____to_____

17	18	19	20	21	22	23	24	25	26	27	28	29	30	31	32	33	34	35

MENSTRUAL FLOW KEY

S = SPOTTING | L = LIGHT | M = MEDIUM | H = HEAVY

Basal Body Temperature Chart

CYCLE DAYS		1	2	3	4	5	6	7	8	9	10	11	12	13	14	15	16
DATE																	
WEEKDAY																	
TIME																	
SEX																	
FLUID																	
FLOW																	
99.	0																
	9																
	8																
	7																
	6																
	5																
98.	4																
	3																
	2																
	1																
	0																
	9																
	8																
	7																
	6																
	5																
97.	4																
	3																
	2																
	1																
	0																
NOTES																	

CERVICAL FLUID KEY

N = NONE | S = STICKY | C = CREAMY | E = EGG WHITE

DATES:_____ to_____

17	18	19	20	21	22	23	24	25	26	27	28	29	30	31	32	33	34	35

MENSTRUAL FLOW KEY

S = SPOTTING | L = LIGHT | M = MEDIUM | H = HEAVY

Basal Body Temperature Chart

CYCLE DAYS		1	2	3	4	5	6	7	8	9	10	11	12	13	14	15	16
DATE																	
WEEKDAY																	
TIME																	
SEX																	
FLUID																	
FLOW																	
99.	0																
	9																
	8																
	7																
	6																
	5																
98.	4																
	3																
	2																
	1																
	0																
	9																
	8																
	7																
	6																
	5																
97.	4																
	3																
	2																
	1																
	0																
NOTES																	

CERVICAL FLUID KEY

N = NONE | S = STICKY | C = CREAMY | E = EGG WHITE

17	18	19	20	21	22	23	24	25	26	27	28	29	30	31	32	33	34	35

MENSTRUAL FLOW KEY

S = SPOTTING | L = LIGHT | M = MEDIUM | H = HEAVY

Basal Body Temperature Chart

CYCLE DAYS		1	2	3	4	5	6	7	8	9	10	11	12	13	14	15	16
DATE																	
WEEKDAY																	
TIME																	
SEX																	
FLUID																	
FLOW																	
99.	0																
	9																
	8																
	7																
	6																
	5																
98.	4																
	3																
	2																
	1																
	0																
	9																
	8																
	7																
	6																
	5																
97.	4																
	3																
	2																
	1																
	0																
NOTES																	

CERVICAL FLUID KEY

N = NONE | S = STICKY | C = CREAMY | E = EGG WHITE

DATES:_____ to_____

	17	18	19	20	21	22	23	24	25	26	27	28	29	30	31	32	33	34	35

MENSTRUAL FLOW KEY

S = SPOTTING | L = LIGHT | M = MEDIUM | H = HEAVY

Basal Body Temperature Chart

CYCLE DAYS		1	2	3	4	5	6	7	8	9	10	11	12	13	14	15	16
DATE																	
WEEKDAY																	
TIME																	
SEX																	
FLUID																	
FLOW																	
99.	0																
	9																
	8																
	7																
	6																
	5																
98.	4																
	3																
	2																
	1																
	0																
	9																
	8																
	7																
	6																
	5																
97.	4																
	3																
	2																
	1																
	0																
NOTES																	

CERVICAL FLUID KEY

N = NONE | S = STICKY | C = CREAMY | E = EGG WHITE

DATES:_____ to_____

17	18	19	20	21	22	23	24	25	26	27	28	29	30	31	32	33	34	35

MENSTRUAL FLOW KEY

S = SPOTTING | L = LIGHT | M = MEDIUM | H = HEAVY

Basal Body Temperature Chart

CYCLE DAYS		1	2	3	4	5	6	7	8	9	10	11	12	13	14	15	16
DATE																	
WEEKDAY																	
TIME																	
SEX																	
FLUID																	
FLOW																	
99.	0																
	9																
	8																
	7																
	6																
	5																
98.	4																
	3																
	2																
	1																
	0																
	9																
	8																
	7																
	6																
	5																
97.	4																
	3																
	2																
	1																
	0																
NOTES																	

CERVICAL FLUID KEY

N = NONE | S = STICKY | C = CREAMY | E = EGG WHITE

17	18	19	20	21	22	23	24	25	26	27	28	29	30	31	32	33	34	35

MENSTRUAL FLOW KEY

S = SPOTTING | L = LIGHT | M = MEDIUM | H = HEAVY

Basal Body Temperature Chart

CYCLE DAYS		1	2	3	4	5	6	7	8	9	10	11	12	13	14	15	16
DATE																	
WEEKDAY																	
TIME																	
SEX																	
FLUID																	
FLOW																	
99.	0																
	9																
	8																
	7																
	6																
	5																
98.	4																
	3																
	2																
	1																
	0																
	9																
	8																
	7																
	6																
	5																
97.	4																
	3																
	2																
	1																
	0																
NOTES																	

CERVICAL FLUID KEY

N = NONE | S = STICKY | C = CREAMY | E = EGG WHITE

DATES:_____ to_____

17	18	19	20	21	22	23	24	25	26	27	28	29	30	31	32	33	34	35

MENSTRUAL FLOW KEY

S = SPOTTING | L = LIGHT | M = MEDIUM | H = HEAVY

Basal Body Temperature Chart

CYCLE DAYS		1	2	3	4	5	6	7	8	9	10	11	12	13	14	15	16
DATE																	
WEEKDAY																	
TIME																	
SEX																	
FLUID																	
FLOW																	
99.	0																
	9																
	8																
	7																
	6																
	5																
98.	4																
	3																
	2																
	1																
	0																
	9																
	8																
	7																
	6																
	5																
97.	4																
	3																
	2																
	1																
	0																
NOTES																	

CERVICAL FLUID KEY

N = NONE | S = STICKY | C = CREAMY | E = EGG WHITE

DATES:_____to_____

17	18	19	20	21	22	23	24	25	26	27	28	29	30	31	32	33	34	35

MENSTRUAL FLOW KEY

S = SPOTTING | L = LIGHT | M = MEDIUM | H = HEAVY

Basal Body Temperature Chart

CYCLE DAYS		1	2	3	4	5	6	7	8	9	10	11	12	13	14	15	16
DATE																	
WEEKDAY																	
TIME																	
SEX																	
FLUID																	
FLOW																	
99.	0																
	9																
	8																
	7																
	6																
	5																
98.	4																
	3																
	2																
	1																
	0																
	9																
	8																
	7																
	6																
	5																
97.	4																
	3																
	2																
	1																
	0																
NOTES																	

CERVICAL FLUID KEY

N = NONE | S = STICKY | C = CREAMY | E = EGG WHITE

17	18	19	20	21	22	23	24	25	26	27	28	29	30	31	32	33	34	35

MENSTRUAL FLOW KEY

S = SPOTTING | L = LIGHT | M = MEDIUM | H = HEAVY

Basal Body Temperature Chart

CYCLE DAYS		1	2	3	4	5	6	7	8	9	10	11	12	13	14	15	16
DATE																	
WEEKDAY																	
TIME																	
SEX																	
FLUID																	
FLOW																	
99.	0																
	9																
	8																
	7																
	6																
	5																
98.	4																
	3																
	2																
	1																
	0																
	9																
	8																
	7																
	6																
	5																
97.	4																
	3																
	2																
	1																
	0																
NOTES																	

CERVICAL FLUID KEY

N = NONE | S = STICKY | C = CREAMY | E = EGG WHITE

DATES:_____ to_____

17	18	19	20	21	22	23	24	25	26	27	28	29	30	31	32	33	34	35

MENSTRUAL FLOW KEY

S = SPOTTING | L = LIGHT | M = MEDIUM | H = HEAVY

Basal Body Temperature Chart

CYCLE DAYS		1	2	3	4	5	6	7	8	9	10	11	12	13	14	15	16
DATE																	
WEEKDAY																	
TIME																	
SEX																	
FLUID																	
FLOW																	
99.	0																
	9																
	8																
	7																
	6																
	5																
98.	4																
	3																
	2																
	1																
	0																
	9																
	8																
	7																
	6																
	5																
97.	4																
	3																
	2																
	1																
	0																
NOTES																	

CERVICAL FLUID KEY

N = NONE | S = STICKY | C = CREAMY | E = EGG WHITE

17	18	19	20	21	22	23	24	25	26	27	28	29	30	31	32	33	34	35

MENSTRUAL FLOW KEY

S = SPOTTING | L = LIGHT | M = MEDIUM | H = HEAVY

Basal Body Temperature Chart

CYCLE DAYS		1	2	3	4	5	6	7	8	9	10	11	12	13	14	15	16
DATE																	
WEEKDAY																	
TIME																	
SEX																	
FLUID																	
FLOW																	
99.	0																
	9																
	8																
	7																
	6																
	5																
98.	4																
	3																
	2																
	1																
	0																
	9																
	8																
	7																
	6																
	5																
97.	4																
	3																
	2																
	1																
	0																
NOTES																	

CERVICAL FLUID KEY

N = NONE | S = STICKY | C = CREAMY | E = EGG WHITE

DATES:_____to_____

17	18	19	20	21	22	23	24	25	26	27	28	29	30	31	32	33	34	35

MENSTRUAL FLOW KEY

S = SPOTTING | L = LIGHT | M = MEDIUM | H = HEAVY

Basal Body Temperature Chart

CYCLE DAYS		1	2	3	4	5	6	7	8	9	10	11	12	13	14	15	16
DATE																	
WEEKDAY																	
TIME																	
SEX																	
FLUID																	
FLOW																	
99.	0																
	9																
	8																
	7																
	6																
	5																
98.	4																
	3																
	2																
	1																
	0																
	9																
	8																
	7																
	6																
	5																
97.	4																
	3																
	2																
	1																
	0																
NOTES																	

CERVICAL FLUID KEY

N = NONE | S = STICKY | C = CREAMY | E = EGG WHITE

DATES:_____to_____

17	18	19	20	21	22	23	24	25	26	27	28	29	30	31	32	33	34	35

MENSTRUAL FLOW KEY

S = SPOTTING | L = LIGHT | M = MEDIUM | H = HEAVY

Chapter 5

Decoding Your Cycle

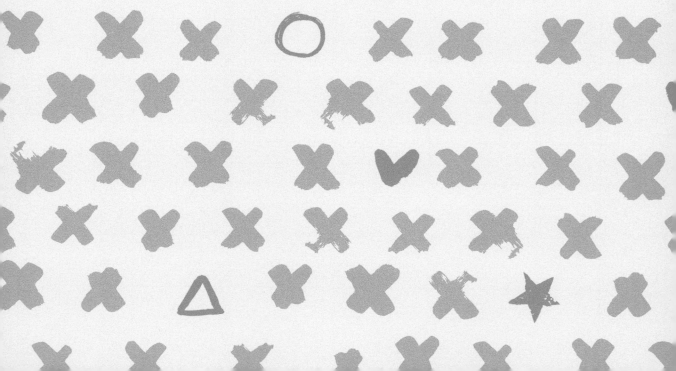

Congratulations on completing your first charts! It's not easy to commit and form new habits, but you did it. Hopefully you are starting to see some patterns emerging in your charts and have been able to make a few connections between the phases of your menstrual cycle and your overall health. For those of you who skipped straight to charting, you may want to take this opportunity to go back and read through the "What You Really Should Know" sections in the earlier chapters to dig deeper into the meaning of your charts.

What You Need and Really Should Know

You've charted your basal body temperature every day as instructed, but what does it all mean? How do you know exactly when you ovulated? Most menstrual cycles have a biphasic temperature shift, meaning there will be a period of time with lower temperatures (follicular phase) followed by a period of time with higher temperatures (luteal phase). Ovulation has occurred when you see a sustained increase in basal body temperature by at least 0.2 degrees Fahrenheit—meaning your temperature goes up at least 0.2 degrees and stays up until your cycle ends. Most women will see a rise of 0.5 degrees to 1 degree, but it can be as subtle as 0.2 degrees and still indicate that ovulation has occurred. If you're having trouble figuring out if you had a temperature rise, you can try charting with a coverline. A coverline is a horizontal line 0.1 degrees above your highest temperature before your temperature rise. If you think you may have had a temperature rise but you're not sure, look back and highlight the last six days of temperatures. Circle the highest of those temperatures and draw a horizontal line 0.1 degrees above that highest temperature. Your luteal phase starts on the day that your temperature rises and stays 0.2 degrees above the horizontal line you've drawn. See the chart on page 89 for an example of a coverline.

Let's take a closer look at your charts. Ask yourself these questions:

- How many days does my menstruation phase usually last?

- Did I have any spotting right before or after my menstruation phase?

- Do I have any days of unexplained spotting during my cycle?

- Have I noticed that my basal body temperature is higher during my menstruation phase?

- How many days is my follicular phase?

- Did I notice a drop in my temperature right before the rise? (That temperature drop is usually on the day of ovulation. Don't worry if you don't have one—not everyone does.)

You are most fertile on the two days prior to ovulation. However, you can get pregnant if you have sex during the five days prior to and the day of ovulation because sperm can live up to five days. You may want to highlight the six days prior to ovulation on each of your charts to make it easier to remember your most fertile days.

Coverline

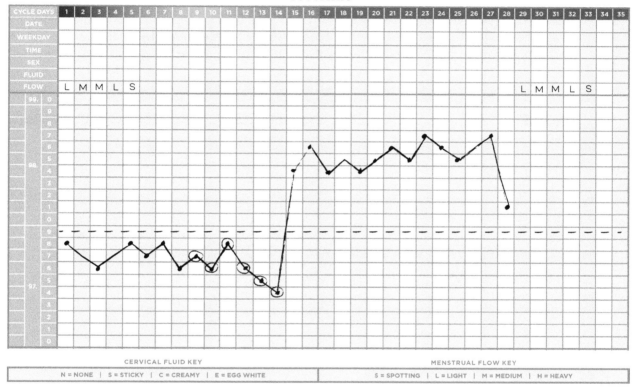

CERVICAL FLUID KEY
N = NONE | S = STICKY | C = CREAMY | E = EGG WHITE

MENSTRUAL FLOW KEY
S = SPOTTING | L = LIGHT | M = MEDIUM | H = HEAVY

A Chart-by-Chart Comparison

Let's take a look at a stereotypically normal chart with a 28-day cycle and a 14-day luteal phase. Note the higher temperature during the menstruation phase, the temperature drop on the day of ovulation, the temperature rise indicating a thermal shift the day after ovulation (the first day of the luteal phase), and the temperature drop the day before the next menstruation phase. Also note the change in cervical fluid from none to sticky to creamy to egg white leading up to ovulation followed by the return to sticky or none after ovulation has occurred. This is a typical cervical fluid pattern in a cycle during which ovulation has occurred.

Average Chart

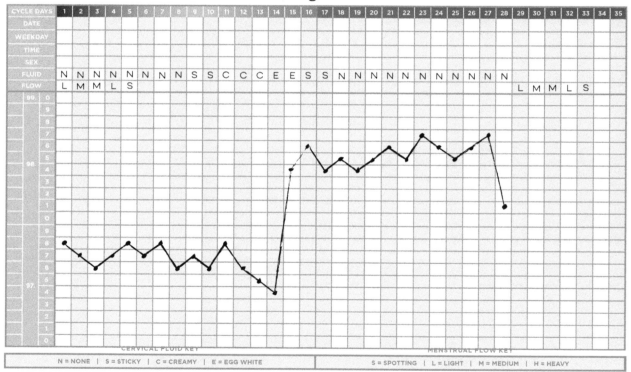

CERVICAL FLUID KEY

N = NONE | S = STICKY | C = CREAMY | E = EGG WHITE

MENSTRUAL FLOW KEY

S = SPOTTING | L = LIGHT | M = MEDIUM | H = HEAVY

Now check out this chart. Notice anything different? Despite a longer-than-average follicular phase, the luteal phase is still within the normal 12- to 16-day range, meaning not only did this woman ovulate, but her corpus luteum produced enough progesterone to have sustained a pregnancy if one had occurred. A long follicular phase can be an indication of low estrogen. Delayed ovulation can also be caused by stress, lack of sleep, low weight or obesity, and certain medications. If you had a particularly stressful month, did you notice your day of ovulation shift later? Your cycle may be longer when you are stressed because the delayed ovulation pushes your 12- to 16-day luteal phase later as well, making your next menstruation phase start later than usual.

Chart with Longer-Than-Average Follicular Phase

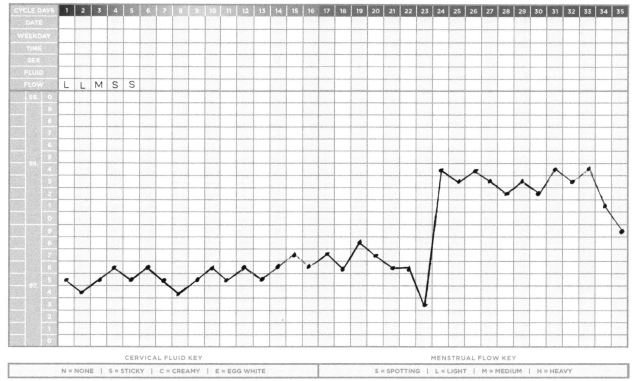

CERVICAL FLUID KEY

N = NONE | S = STICKY | C = CREAMY | E = EGG WHITE

MENSTRUAL FLOW KEY

S = SPOTTING | L = LIGHT | M = MEDIUM | H = HEAVY

Does your chart look more or less like the standard charts in this book? If so, you can skip directly to the Resources section of the book. If you have a chart that is out of the ordinary, read on to chapter 6, where we will explore the medical conditions, lifestyle choices, and medications that might be making your charts more difficult to understand.

CHART CHEAT SHEET

- Spotting before your menstruation phase after at least 10 days of high temperatures can be normal. However, if the temperature rise lasts less than 10 days, spotting could indicate a premature breakdown of the corpus luteum and a short luteal phase.

- Very light periods can indicate an anovulatory cycle or an insufficient endometrial lining. Check your chart for signs of ovulation that cycle.

- Mid-cycle spotting around the time of ovulation is normal and is a result of an estrogen drop immediately before ovulation. Spotting that lasts more than a day or two or does not happen near ovulation may indicate an issue like polyps or a sexually transmitted infection.

- If you have a fever, continue to chart your temperature, but make a note of it so you don't mistake your fever temperature increase for your thermal shift.

- If you have 18 or more high temperatures after ovulation, you might be pregnant, or you might have an ovarian cyst. Now is a good time to take a pregnancy test.

- Spotting after sex occurs most often after ovulation when the cervix is at its lowest. Spotting after sex can be caused by sexually transmitted infections, an inflammation of the cervix called cervicitis, or cervical polyps. Make an appointment with a health care provider just to be safe.

- If you have erratic temperatures and your chart really doesn't make any sense, it's time to troubleshoot. If you are using a digital thermometer, check the batteries or try switching to glass. If you're using glass, make sure you take your temperature for the entire five minutes and consider taking your temperature vaginally rather than orally. Make sure you are taking your temperature at exactly the same time every day. If you do take it at a different time, make note of it.

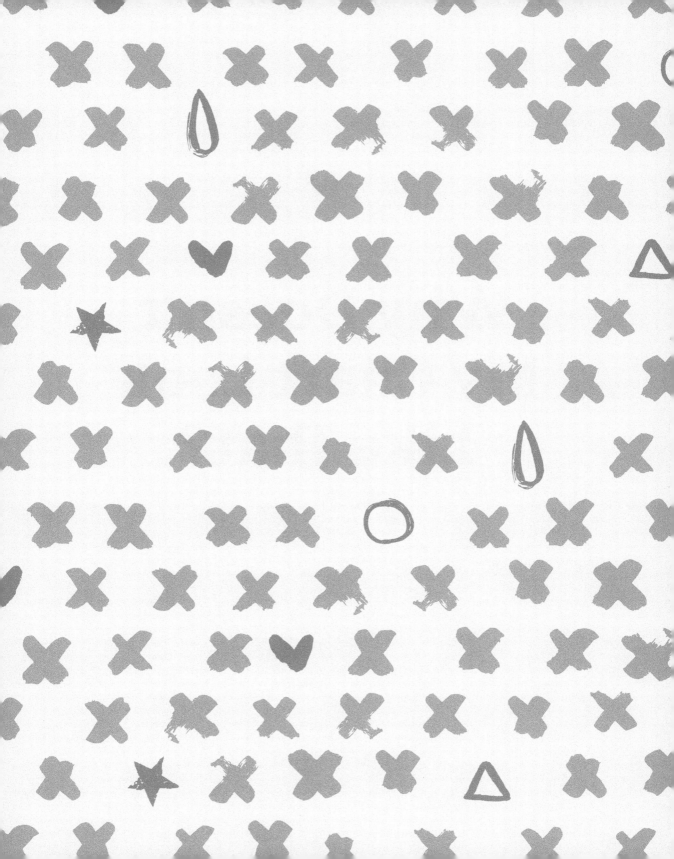

Chapter 6

Why Doesn't My Chart Look Like That?

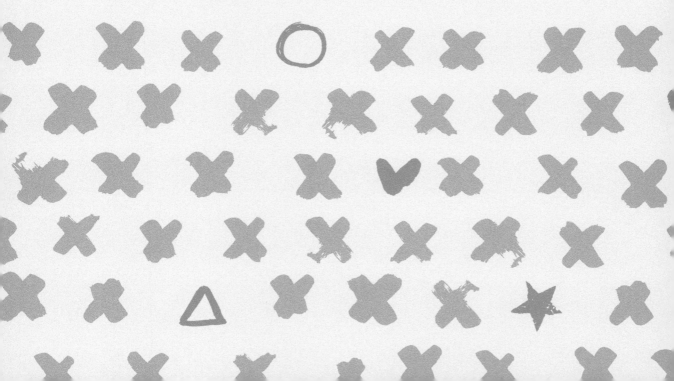

You did it! You finished your charts. You woke up every morning, took your temperature, identified your cervical fluid, and charted it all. Now it's time to put it all together and figure out what your cycle is telling you about how to improve your health.

What You Need to Know

So what does it mean if your chart doesn't match any of the sample charts in chapter 4 of this book? It could mean that you have a common medical, hormonal, or lifestyle imbalance that needs to be evaluated.

PCOS

Polycystic ovary syndrome (PCOS) is a hormonal disorder that is thought to affect 6 percent to 15 percent of women of childbearing age. It is the most common cause of infertility in women. It's unclear what causes PCOS, but according to a prospective study published in the *Journal of Pediatric Endocrinology and Metabolism*, 35 percent of mothers and 40 percent of sisters of patients with PCOS are also affected by PCOS themselves, implying that there is a genetic component to PCOS. According to the 2003 Rotterdam Consesus Criteria, women must have two of the three following criteria to be diagnosed with PCOS: oligo-ovulation or anovulation, clinical and/or biochemical signs, and hyperandrogenism or polycystic ovaries.

Endometriosis

Endometriosis is a medical condition where the lining of the uterus grows in areas of your body other than the uterus. Endometriosis occurs in 1 in 10 women and is most often diagnosed in women in their 30s and 40s. A woman is more likely to develop endometriosis if she is underweight and if she started her period before age 11. She is at a sixfold increased risk of having endometriosis if her mother, sister, or aunt has endometriosis.

The endometrial tissue outside the uterus responds to estrogen levels the same way the endometrial tissue inside the uterus does: It grows, breaks down, and bleeds with each menstrual cycle. This growing and bleeding causes inflammation and irritation of the surrounding tissues and organs, which can lead to the formation of scar tissue or adhesions. The scar tissue and adhesions cause the pain associated with endometriosis. The most common locations to find endometriosis are the ovaries, the fallopian tubes, the ligaments that hold the uterus in place, or the outer surface of the uterus. However, endometriosis can grow anywhere and has even been found in the lungs, brain, and skin.

Women with endometriosis have severely painful menstrual cramps during their periods, chronic pelvic pain, pain while having bowel movements or urinating during their periods, and pain during or after sex. Women with endometriosis usually have shorter menstrual cycles (shorter than 27 days) with a menstruation phase longer than seven days and may have spotting between periods.

Endometriosis

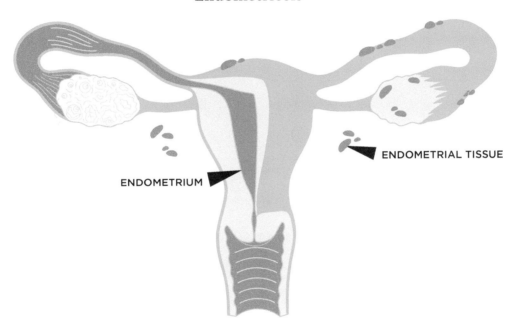

ENDOMETRIUM

ENDOMETRIAL TISSUE

Uterine Growths

Any abnormality of the uterus can affect your menstrual cycle. The two most common growths inside the uterus are fibroids (also known as leiomyomas or myomas) and polyps.

Fibroids are benign smooth tissue growths inside or on the walls of the uterus and can range in size from a seed to a grapefruit or even larger. According to the United States Department of Health and Human Services, fibroids are most common in women between 35 and 50 years old, African American women, obese women, and women with a family history of fibroids. Although 20 percent to 80 percent of women develop fibroids in their lifetime, most are asymptomatic, so most women don't even know they have them. Women who do have symptomatic fibroids often have heavy and extended periods of menstrual bleeding with clots and pelvic pain.

Fibroids

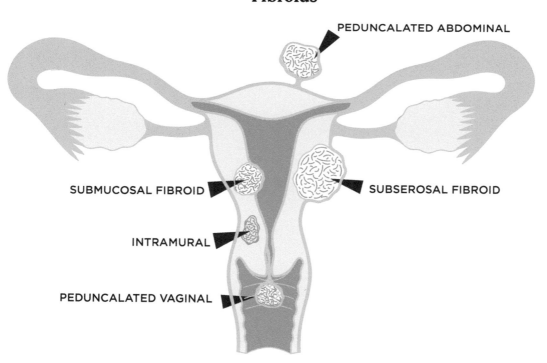

Uterine polyps are small overgrowths of the endometrium (the lining of the uterus). Polyps can be as small as a sesame seed or grow to be as large as a golf ball. They can grow within the uterus or protrude through the cervix. Polyps are most likely to occur in women who are in perimenopause (the years prior to menopause) or are in menopause. They are usually benign but can also be precancerous or cancerous. Polyps can cause spotting between periods, spotting after sex, heavy bleeding during periods, and bleeding after menopause.

Polyps

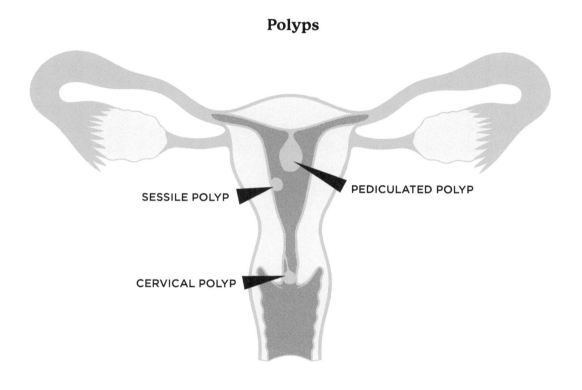

SESSILE POLYP

PEDICULATED POLYP

CERVICAL POLYP

Hormone Imbalance

Your body is literally controlled by the hormones of the endocrine system. Glands release hormones that act as messengers between your organs. When the body releases too many or too few of these hormones, your organs get mixed messages, leading to issues with sleep, mood, metabolism, stress, and your menstrual cycle. The hormones most likely to affect your menstrual cycle are secreted by the adrenal glands, thyroid, pancreas, and ovaries. The longer these hormones are out of balance, the harder they can be to fix.

The adrenal glands secrete cortisol and adrenal androgens (DHEA and testosterone). An imbalance of adrenal hormones can cause feelings of anxiety, weight gain or difficulty losing weight, acne, and excessive hair growth or hair loss. An imbalance of thyroid hormones can cause you to feel restless or tired, have thin or brittle hair and nails, and gain or lose weight, and it can cause your periods to be very heavy or to stop altogether. Too much or too little thyroid hormone can also delay ovulation. The pancreas secretes the hormone insulin, but for some women the insulin secreted cannot be absorbed by the body (also known as insulin resistance). Excess insulin inhibits ovulation and stimulates the ovaries to produce more testosterone. Women with type 1 diabetes tend to have longer, heavier periods, whereas women with type 2 diabetes tend to have longer overall cycles.

Lifestyle

Chronic stress, poor diet, medications, and lack of sleep can all cause irregular menstrual cycles. Stress can increase cortisol levels, which can suppress ovulation. Weight gain and weight loss can have a positive or negative affect on your menstrual cycle, depending on your starting weight. A woman with a healthy BMI who exercises or diets excessively and loses weight may experience suppressed ovulation and irregular menstrual cycles. Conversely, a woman who is overweight or obese may be able to regulate her menstrual cycle by gradually losing weight, though that may require a woman to pinpoint and address other related health abnormalities. Any medication that works by controlling different hormones will also likely affect your menstrual cycle. Some examples are thyroid medications, birth control pills, antipsychotic medications, some tricyclic antidepressants, and seizure medications. Even NSAIDs, a class of drugs often used to help with menstrual cramps, can impair the menstrual cycle.

What You Really Should Know

Wait, do I have any of those things? I don't know, but your charts can help! Let's take a look.

PCOS

PCOS is a hormonal disorder characterized by oligo-ovulation or anovulation, clinical and/or biochemical signs, and hyperandrogenism or polycystic ovaries. That's super clear, right? Yeah, it's not clear to health care providers either. In fact, most women see three or more health care providers over the span of two or more years before they are diagnosed with PCOS. This is particularly unfortunate because early diagnosis and intervention are extremely important to improve the health and quality of life for women with PCOS. The most common symptoms of PCOS are irregular periods, excessive hair growth, acne, thinning hair or baldness, obesity or difficulty losing weight, and darkening of the skin. Though some women with PCOS are obese, it is also common to have lean PCOS (PCOS without obesity). Women with PCOS are more likely to develop diabetes, cardiovascular disease, and endometrial cancer.

Let's break down the diagnostic criteria.

Oligo-ovulation or anovulation: Women with PCOS have irregular or absent periods. If they do have periods, they might have fewer than eight menstrual cycles per year or cycles longer than 35 days.

Clinical and/or biochemical markers of PCOS: Women with PCOS produce excess androgenic hormones. Excess androgenic hormones make women with PCOS more prone to acne, hirsutism (excessive body hair growth), and baldness. Women with PCOS also have high levels of insulin due to insulin resistance. Insulin resistance is especially common in women who are obese, do not get enough physical activity, have unhealthy eating habits, or have a family history of type 2 diabetes.

Polycystic ovaries: Polycystic means many cysts. In women with PCOS, multiple fluid-filled cysts develop in the ovaries. These fluid-filled sacs are actually follicles containing immature eggs that, due to the hormone imbalances present in PCOS, never mature enough to trigger ovulation. These cysts continue to grow, causing multiple cysts that appear like a string of pearls on an ultrasound. Although you may think ovarian cysts are the clearest sign of PCOS (those cysts are literally the name of the disorder), up to 62 percent of women without PCOS also have cysts on their ovaries. Due to this, a diagnosis of PCOS cannot be made without meeting at least one of the other criteria.

Women with PCOS will likely have a chart that shows a menstrual cycle longer than 35 days in which ovulation may or may not occur. They often have higher-than-normal levels of estrogen. This makes their cervical fluid consistently watery with an egg white consistency throughout their cycles as opposed to only during ovulation.

You might be thinking, "So you're telling me that if I have PCOS, I may chart forever without seeing a thermal shift or a change in cervical fluid? Why am I doing this again?" To this I say: Because you just figured out you have PCOS. Remember when I said most women take at least two years to be diagnosed with PCOS? That's because in order to be diagnosed with PCOS, women need to get sonograms, chart their periods, and do blood tests to confirm whether they are ovulating. If you have been charting your temperatures and cervical fluid, you can deliver the proof in your charts. Your charts will show your health care provider that your cycles are longer than 35 days, that you are having fewer than eight menstrual cycles per year, or that you aren't ovulating. In this case, the only thing the health care provider needs to do is check with you to see if you have the physical signs of PCOS or do a sonogram to look for cysts. Then, you'll have your answer! You just saved yourself two years of testing and doctor visits.

The good news is that if you're not trying to get pregnant, treatment for PCOS can be very simple. Hormonal birth control methods regulate your hormones and prevent the dangerous effects of irregular or absent periods. If you are trying to get pregnant, things can get slightly more complicated but not at all impossible. If you're in this boat, there are some support groups and forums listed in the Resources section at the end of this book.

PCOS Chart

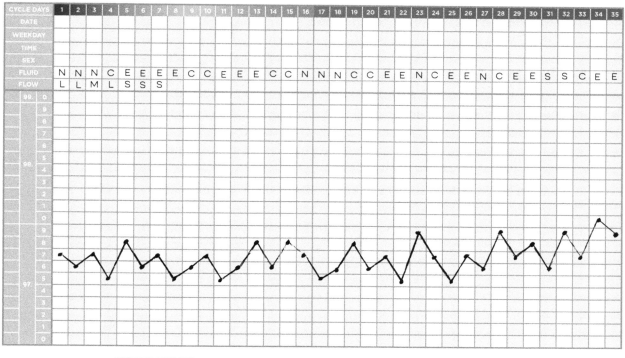

CYCLE DAYS	1	2	3	4	5	6	7	8	9	10	11	12	13	14	15	16	17	18	19	20	21	22	23	24	25	26	27	28	29	30	31	32	33	34	35
DATE																																			
WEEKDAY																																			
TIME																																			
SEX																																			
FLUID	N	N	C	E	E	E	E	C	C	E	E	E	C	N	N	C	C	E	E	N	C	E	E	N	C	E	E	S	S	C	E	E			
FLOW	L	L	M	L	S	S	S																												

CERVICAL FLUID KEY

N = NONE | S = STICKY | C = CREAMY | E = EGG WHITE

MENSTRUAL FLOW KEY

S = SPOTTING | L = LIGHT | M = MEDIUM | H = HEAVY

Endometriosis

Endometriosis is a medical condition where the interior lining of the uterus also grows outside the uterus. The American College of Obstetricians and Gynecologists estimates that 1 in 10 women have endometriosis and that 30 percent to 40 percent of women with endometriosis will experience infertility. The most common symptom of endometriosis is pelvic pain, usually associated with menstruation. This pain is much worse than average and usually increases the longer you have endometriosis. There are a variety of other signs and symptoms of endometriosis such as pain during or after sex, pain with bowel movements, excessively heavy bleeding or bleeding between periods, fatigue, diarrhea, constipation, bloating, nausea, and infertility.

Since there are so many symptoms for endometriosis, it can be hard to diagnose. Endometriosis can be misdiagnosed as conditions that cause similar symptoms, such as ovarian cysts and irritable bowel syndrome (IBS). There are a few different ways a health care provider can check if you have endometriosis. One way is through a physical exam where it's possible, although unlikely, to feel the scar tissue of endometriosis. Another way is to look at a sonogram where it's possible to see the cysts associated with endometriosis (endometriomas) but unlikely to see endometriosis itself. There is also laparoscopy, a surgical procedure in which a small camera is inserted into your abdomen to look for endometriosis. If it is found, your doctor can do a small biopsy of the tissue to officially determine whether or not you have endometriosis. That all sounds like a fun adventure, right? I don't think so, either. According to the Endometriosis Foundation of America, the average time it takes a woman to be diagnosed with endometriosis is 10 years. TEN YEARS! This delay in diagnosis and treatment is especially detrimental since the longer you have untreated endometriosis, the more damage it can do to your body.

Charting can help you identify the signs of endometriosis so you can start treatment sooner. Treating the symptoms of endometriosis can be as simple as using hormonal contraception, but treatment of the disease usually involves surgery. Women with endometriosis have more tissue to shed, so they usually have a menstruation phase longer than seven days with brown spotting at the end of the phase. They may experience bleeding or pain during ovulation, and their cycle length is often shorter than 28 days. Women with endometriosis may notice a temperature greater that 97.8 degrees on the first three days of the menstruation phase with no premenstrual temperature drop. They may also see a drop in basal body temperature during the early follicular phase. Women with endometriosis usually have little to no cervical fluid.

Endometriosis Chart

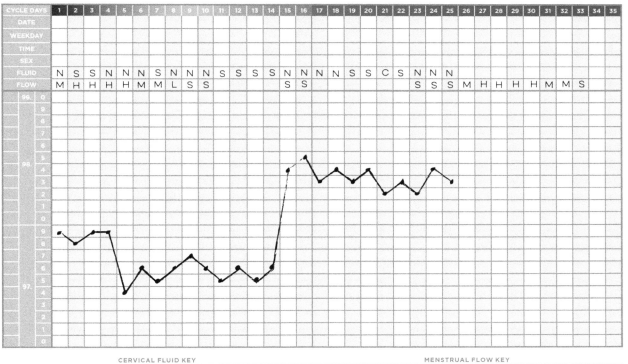

Uterine Growths

The two most common growths inside the uterus are fibroids (also known as leiomyomas or myomas) and polyps. Fibroids are benign smooth tissue growths inside or on the walls of the uterus and can range in size from a seed to a grapefruit or even larger. Uterine polyps are small overgrowths of the endometrium (the lining of the uterus). Polyps can be as small as a sesame seed or grow to be as large as a golf ball. They can grow within or protrude through the cervix.

Both fibroids and polyps are estrogen sensitive, meaning they grow during times of increased estrogen, and can be associated with infertility. Both fibroids

Fibroid Chart

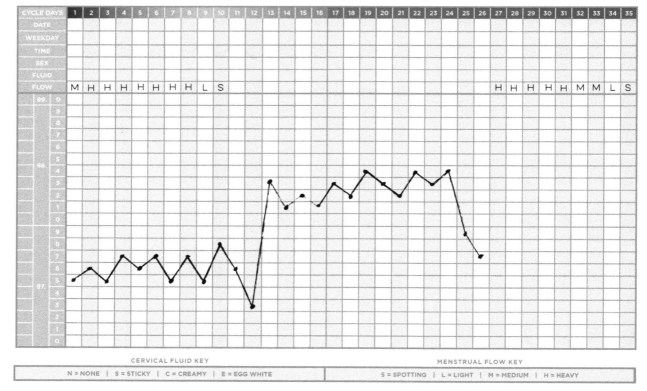

CERVICAL FLUID KEY	MENSTRUAL FLOW KEY
N = NONE | S = STICKY | C = CREAMY | E = EGG WHITE	S = SPOTTING | L = LIGHT | M = MEDIUM | H = HEAVY

and polyps can be diagnosed with a pelvic exam and/or pelvic sonogram. Since fibroids are estrogen sensitive, treatment options include progesterone-only contraception, such as a hormonal IUD, implant, injection, or pills, or surgical management. Women who have cervical polyps can have them removed in a pain-less office procedure, whereas women who have endometrial polyps may need a more in-depth procedure.

Women who have fibroids often have heavy and extended periods of menstrual bleeding with clots and pelvic pain. Polyps can cause spotting between periods and after sex, heavy bleeding during periods, and bleeding after menopause.

Polyps Chart

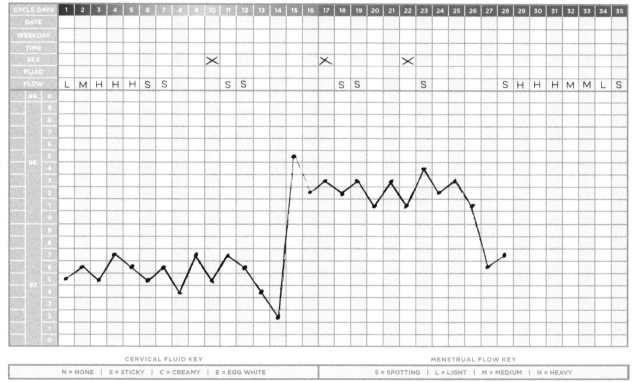

CERVICAL FLUID KEY

N = NONE | S = STICKY | C = CREAMY | E = EGG WHITE

MENSTRUAL FLOW KEY

S = SPOTTING | L = LIGHT | M = MEDIUM | H = HEAVY

Hormone Imbalance

Hormones coordinate everything from sleep to growth to pregnancy and, of course, your menstrual cycle. The hormones most likely to affect your menstrual cycle are secreted by the adrenal glands, thyroid, pancreas, and ovaries.

ADRENAL GLANDS

The adrenal glands secrete cortisol, adrenal androgens, DHEA (the precursor to estrogen), and testosterone. They secrete cortisol as a response to stress. When you experience chronic stress, the adrenal glands produce more cortisol and, as a result, produce less of the hormones you need to control your menstrual cycle. High cortisol levels lead to long menstrual cycles because not enough DHEA (and the resulting estrogen) is produced to trigger ovulation. On your chart, you will notice a longer-than-average follicular phase and an absent or a late thermal shift, indicating anovulation. You may also notice spotting during your luteal phase or a shorter luteal phase as a result of the cortisol suppressing progesterone production.

Cortisol Chart

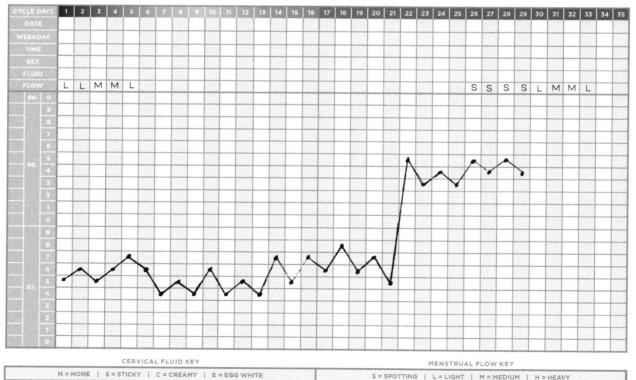

THYROID

Your thyroid plays a big role in helping to control your menstrual cycle. Disruptions in normal thyroid hormones can lower progesterone. Too much thyroid hormone (hyperthyroidism) or too little thyroid hormone (hypothyroidism) can make your periods very light, very heavy, irregular, or nonexistent. Pretty much anything goes. Helpful right? Since there is no "typical" menstrual cycle with thyroid disorders, basal body temperature and cervical fluid charting is particularly helpful in identifying these medical conditions. One of the most common chart patterns of a thyroid condition is the difference in basal body temperatures throughout all phases of the menstrual cycle. Most pre-ovulatory basal body temperatures are between 97.0 and 97.7 degrees and most post-ovulatory basal body temperatures are higher than 97.8 degrees. If you have hyperthyroidism, you'll have a higher-than-average basal body temperature, long cycles, and very light periods. If you have hypothyroidism, you'll have a lower-than-average basal body temperature, long cycles, and heavy periods with anovulation (no thermal shift). Women with hypothyroidism may also have prolonged, wet, slippery cervical fluid.

Hyperthyroid Chart

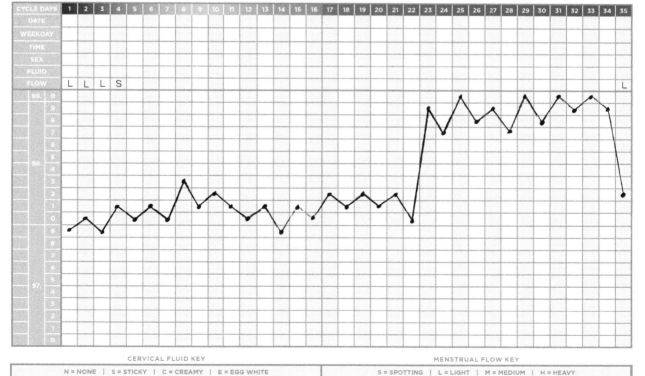

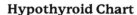

Hypothyroid Chart

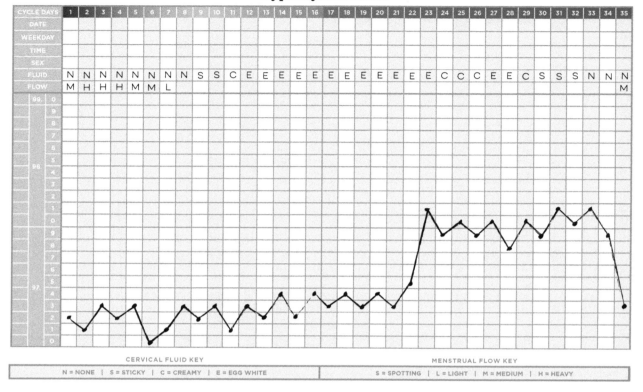

CYCLE DAYS	1	2	3	4	5	6	7	8	9	10	11	12	13	14	15	16	17	18	19	20	21	22	23	24	25	26	27	28	29	30	31	32	33	34	35
DATE																																			
WEEKDAY																																			
TIME																																			
SEX																																			
FLUID	N	N	N	N	N	N	N	S	S	C	E	E	E	E	E	E	E	E	E	E	E	E	C	C	C	E	E	C	S	S	N	N	N
FLOW	M	H	H	H	M	M	L																												M

CERVICAL FLUID KEY
N = NONE | S = STICKY | C = CREAMY | E = EGG WHITE

MENSTRUAL FLOW KEY
S = SPOTTING | L = LIGHT | M = MEDIUM | H = HEAVY

PANCREAS AND OVARIES

The pancreas secretes the hormone insulin, but some women's bodies continue to reject the insulin (also known as insulin resistance), resulting in an excess of the hormone. Insulin resistance occurs in up to 95 percent of women with obese PCOS and 75 percent of women with lean PCOS. We know that insulin resistance and infertility are closely linked to PCOS, but does insulin resistance cause PCOS and infertility or does PCOS and infertility cause insulin resistance? The answer is it's probably both, and it's probably cyclic. Excess insulin lowers FSH and LH, the hormones that trigger a follicle to mature and release an egg from the ovary at ovulation. This delays or stops ovulation, which then causes the ovaries to produce more testosterone, one of the biochemical markers used to diagnose PCOS. See? It's all linked.

Women with insulin resistance will have a chart similar to women with PCOS: longer cycles with delayed or absent ovulation.

Please see the PCOS chart on page 103 for an example of what this chart may look like.

Lifestyle

Many women believe that their stress causes a late menstruation phase. Though it may feel that way, excess stress can only affect the follicular phase, thus delaying ovulation, not menstruation. Yes, your period is late, but it's not because of stress that's happening now, but rather from the stress that happened more than 12 to 16 days prior. Even though stress in the luteal phase cannot stop a post-ovulatory period from coming, it can cause spotting before that period or cause an early period. This happens because stress produces cortisol, and cortisol uses progesterone. As we learned earlier in this book, our luteal phase lasts until our progesterone levels drop. Increased cortisol causes them to drop before they naturally would. Women with chronic stress may have charts that show a longer-than-average follicular phase and delayed ovulation. If the cortisol is suppressing the progesterone production, you'll get a shorter-than-average luteal phase and spotting before the menstruation phase.

Please see the high cortisol chart on page 108 for an example of what this chart may look like.

WEIGHT

Weight gain and weight loss can have a positive or negative effect on your menstrual cycle, depending on your starting weight. A woman with a normal BMI who loses weight by excessively exercising or dieting may experience suppressed ovulation and irregular menstrual cycles. This is because your body needs a certain amount of fat to produce the estrogen needed to stimulate ovulation. Just as too little fat can suppress ovulation because of low estrogen, women with high levels of fat can have too much estrogen, which can also suppress ovulation. A woman with a high BMI who loses even 5 percent of her body weight can actually lower her estrogen levels stored in body fat enough to start ovulating regularly. Women who are obese (BMI greater than 30) or underweight (BMI less than 18.5) may have charts that show signs of anovulation, irregular or infrequent menstrual cycles, and very light (underweight) or heavy (overweight) periods.

Underweight Chart

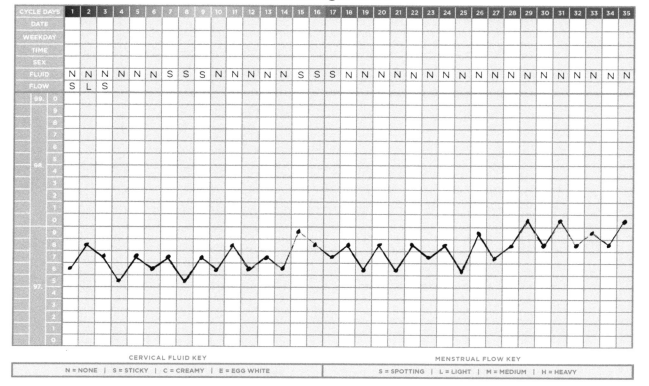

CYCLE DAYS	1	2	3	4	5	6	7	8	9	10	11	12	13	14	15	16	17	18	19	20	21	22	23	24	25	26	27	28	29	30	31	32	33	34	35
DATE																																			
WEEKDAY																																			
TIME																																			
SEX																																			
FLUID	N	N	N	N	N	N	S	S	S	N	N	N	N	N	S	S	S	N	N	N	N	N	N	N	N	N	N	N	N	N	N	N	N	N	N
FLOW	S	L	S																																

CERVICAL FLUID KEY
N = NONE | S = STICKY | C = CREAMY | E = EGG WHITE

MENSTRUAL FLOW KEY
S = SPOTTING | L = LIGHT | M = MEDIUM | H = HEAVY

NSAIDS

Drugs like hormonal birth control are known to affect your menstrual cycle. Other classes of drugs, such as tricyclic antidepressants, thyroid medications, and seizure medications, might also affect it. An even more surprising class of drug that can affect your menstrual cycle includes NSAIDs. NSAIDs are pain medications often used to help painful periods, but they can also reduce the amount of bleeding during a period as well. In fact, health care providers often prescribe NSAIDs to women who suffer from excessive bleeding during their periods. Even though this seems like a win-win situation, studies have shown that NSAIDs can actually inhibit ovulation. Follicles in the ovaries release prostaglandins in response to the LH surge (the surge of hormones that triggers ovulation). NSAIDs work by blocking prostaglandins, so if you take NSAIDs regularly, they could be preventing ovulation.

Please see the underweight chart in the previous section and the PCOS chart on page 103 for examples of anovulatory cycles.

HOW CAN I RELATE?

Meet Becca. Becca has been charting for years, but when she first started, she admits she was lost.

My periods have always been irregular. I knew that I got my period every once in a while, but I didn't know when to expect it or why these irregular periods were happening. I had regular periods while taking birth control pills, but whenever I went off of them, my period would become crazy irregular again. When I first started, my charts were all over the place. For months, I waited to see a pattern, for any sign of anything repetitive from chart to chart. It took a while, but I finally started to see that the clues to my health issues were actually in the lack of patterns in my charts. I was able to bring my charts to my midwife, and together, we figured out that I have a hormonal imbalance called PCOS that was causing my irregular periods. I love charting because I can finally tell when I'm ovulating and when to expect my period. I finally have an answer to why my periods are the way they are.

What's Next?

You should be so proud of yourself! You committed to learning more about your body, health, and menstrual cycle. You took your temperature every morning, checked your cervical fluid, and charted every day. You read and learned about your menstrual cycle and what it's trying to tell you about your overall health and well-being. You may have even identified some irregularities. So, now what? Bring your chart to your health care provider! Remember, most of the syndromes and conditions we learned about can take years to diagnose because your health care provider usually has to start the investigation from scratch. By bringing them evidence of your menstrual cycle irregularities, you've just given yourself a huge head start to get your diagnosis.

Okay. Let's be real for a second. Not every health care provider is going to want to hear about your charts. In fact, some may brush them off, dismiss your symptoms, and expect you to simply do as they say. Some others may think they know how to interpret your charts and how to treat your symptoms, but in reality, they're just following an algorithm and not treating your individual symptoms and needs.

You know better than that! You know your body, and you know better than to let someone dismiss you simply because they have the degree. You know you deserve to be heard. Now is the time to trust your instincts and find a provider who listens to and is willing to work with you. If you aren't getting a helpful response from your health care provider, it may be time to find a new one. Talk to your friends. Take to the blogs. Check the Resources section at the end of this book. See if there is a health care provider in your area whom other people using the fertility awareness method have liked and felt supported by. This provider may be a specialist like an endocrinologist, a reproductive endocrinologist, a midwife, a homeopath, or a family medicine doctor. Remember: There is no perfect provider except for the provider who is perfect for you!

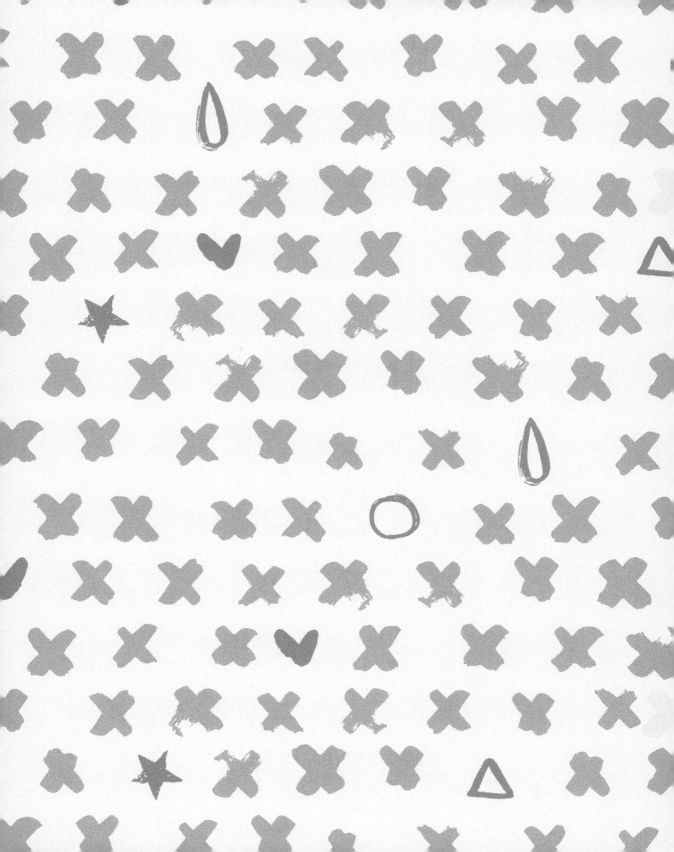

Conclusion

Thank you for exploring the fertility awareness method with me. I hope that you have found this book fun to read and full of useful information. You have all the tools you need to chart your cycle, decipher what it's telling you about your overall health, and take the next steps to fix what might be broken. You should now be able to identify the phases of your menstrual cycle and to determine whether they are typical or irregular. You should understand more about what different irregularities mean and know whether you can make changes to help yourself or you should seek medical attention. Happy charting!

Resources

Support and Forums

EndoMetropolis (Facebook Group)
www.facebook.com/groups/endometropolis/

Fertility Awareness Method of Birth Control (Facebook Group)
wwww.facebook.com/groups/FertilityAwareness.BirthControl/

How to Choose a Psychologist on the American Psychological Association website
www.apa.org/helpcenter/choose-therapist.aspx

PCOS on Supportgroups
pcos.supportgroups.com

r/Fertility Awareness Method on Reddit
www.reddit.com/r/PCOS/

"Trying to Get Pregnant" on The Bump Forums
forums.thebump.com/discussion/12727707/
fertility-awareness-charting-and-low-temperature

Fertility

Fertility Awareness Center
www.fertaware.com/

Infertility Network
www.infertilitynetwork.org

RESOLVE: The National Infertility Association
resolve.org

Taking Charge of Your Fertility
www.tcoyf.com

PCOS

American Thyroid Association
   www.thyroid.org

"How to Reduce the Damaging Effects of PCOS on Fertility Through Diet
   and Herbs"
   natural-fertility-info.com/pcos-fertility-diet

PCOS Awareness Association
   www.pcosaa.org

Soul Cysters
   soulcysters.com

Endometriosis

Endo Warriors
   endowarriorssupport.com

Endo What?
   www.EndoWhat.com

Endometriosis Foundation of America
   www.endofound.org

References

American College of Obstetricians and Gynecologists. "Endometriosis FAQ." January 2019. https://www.acog.org/~/media/For%20Patients/faq013.pdf?dmc=1&ts =20130407T1941277956.

American Pregnancy Association. "Cervical Mucus and Your Fertility." Accessed May 14, 2019. https://americanpregnancy.org/getting-pregnant/cervical-mucus.

American Pregnancy Association. "Understanding Ovulation." Last modified May 14, 2019. https://americanpregnancy.org/getting-pregnant/understanding-ovulation.

Azziz, R., and M. D. Kashar-Miller. "Family History as a Risk Factor for the Polycystic Ovary Syndrome." *Journal of Pediatric Endocrinology and Metabolism* 13, Supplement 5 (2000): 1303–1306.

Boutot, Maegan. "Stress and the Menstrual Cycle." *Clue.* November 9, 2016. https:// helloclue.com/articles/cycle-a-z/stress-your-period.

Briden, Lara. "The Link Between PCOS and Insulin Resistance." *Clue.* September 3, 2018. https://helloclue.com/articles/cycle-a-z/the-link-between-pcos-and-insulin -resistance.

Centers for Disease Control and Prevention. "Birth Control Methods." Last modified December 3, 2018. https://www.cdc.gov/reproductivehealth/contraception /index.htm.

Chai, Sungji, and Robert A. Wild. "Basal Body Temperature and Endometriosis." *Fertility and Sterility* 54, no. 6 (December 1990): 1028–1031. doi:10.1016 /S0015-0282(16)54000-X.

Chiazze, Leonard, Jr., Franklin T. Brayer, John J. Macisco Jr., Margaret P. Parker, and Benedict J. Duffy. "The Length and Variability of the Human Menstrual Cycle." *Journal of the American Medical Association* 203, no. 6 (February 5, 1968): 377–380. doi:10.1001/jama.1968.03140060001001.

Chisholm, Andrea. "Can a Weight Change Affect Your Period? How a Sudden Drop or Increase Affects Your Cycle." Last modified May 18, 2019. https://www.verywellhealth.com/changes-in-your-weight-and-missing-your-period-4105209.

Clue. "The Myth of Moon Phases and Menstruation." Last modified April 16, 2019. https://helloclue.com/articles/cycle-a-z/myth-moon-phases-menstruation.

Coughlin, Sara. "9 Period Euphemisms from Around the World." *Refinery29*. May 4, 2016. https://www.refinery29.com/en-us/period-menstrual-cycle-slang-words-translations.

Cunningham, F. Gary, Kenneth J. Leveno, Steven L. Bloom, Catherine Y. Spong, Jodi S. Dashe, Barbara L. Hoffman, Brian M. Casey, and Jeanne S. Sheffield. *Williams Obstetrics*. 24th ed. New York: McGraw-Hill Education, 2014.

Cutler, Winnifred B. "Lunar and Menstrual Phase Locking." *American Journal of Obstetrics and Gynecology* 137, no. 7 (August 1980): 834–839. doi:10.1016/0002-9378(80)90895-9.

Crawford, Natalie M., David A. Pritchard, Amy H. Herring, and Anne Z. Steiner. "Prospective Evaluation of Luteal Phase Length and Natural Fertility." *Fertility and Sterility* 107, no. 3 (March 2017): 749–755. doi:10.1016/j.fertnstert.2016.11.022.

Davis, Joseph B., and James H. Segars. "Menstruation and Menstrual Disorders: Anovulation." *Global Library of Women's Medicine*. Last modified May 2009. https://www.glowm.com/section_view/item/295.

Eisinger, Steve. "Uterine Fibroids." *Office on Women's Health*. Last modified April 1, 2019. https://www.womenshealth.gov/a-z-topics/uterine-fibroids.

Endometriosis Foundation of America. "What Is Endometriosis? Causes, Symptoms, and Treatments." Accessed July 31, 2019. https://www.endofound.org/endometriosis.

Fauser, Bart C.J.M. et al. "Consensus on Women's Health Aspects of Polycystic Ovary Syndrome (PCOS): The Amsterdam ESHRE/ASRM-Sponsored 3rd PCOS Consensus Workshop Group." *Fertility and Sterility* 97, no. 1 (January 2012): 28–38. doi:10.1016/j.fertnstert.2011.09.024.

Gnoth, C., D. Godehardt, E. Godehardt, P. Frank-Hermann, and G. Freundl. "Time to Pregnancy: Results of the German Prospective Study and Impact on the Management of Infertility." *Human Reproduction* 18, no. 9 (September 2003): 1959–1966. doi:10.1093/humrep/deg366.

Gurevich, Rachel. "What to Know Before You Buy a Basal Body Thermometer." *Very Well Family*. Last modified May 1, 2019. https://www.verywellfamily.com /before-you-buy-a-basal-body-temperature-thermometer-1960283.

Hatcher, Robert A. *Contraceptive Technology*. New York: Ardent Media, 2004.

Higuera, Valencia. "Short Luteal Phase: Causes, Symptoms, and Treatment." *Healthline*. Last modified May 10, 2017. https://www.healthline.com/health/pregnancy /short-luteal-phase.

Hutchins, Jessica. "Your Blood Sugar May Be the Key to Your Hormone Imbalance." *Cleveland Clinic*. November 11, 2015. https://health.clevelandclinic.org /polycystic-ovary-syndrome-pill-not-remedy.

Klepchukova, Anna. "Chemical Pregnancy: Symptoms, Causes, and Prevention of Miscarriage." *Flo Health*. Last modified January 2, 2019. https://flo.health /pregnancy/pregnancy-health/pregnancy-loss/chemical-pregnancy.

Klepchukova, Anna. "Hormonal Imbalance in Women: 9 Signs You Have It." *Flo Health*. Last modified January 4, 2019. https://flo.health/menstrual-cycle/health /symptoms-and-diseases/hormonal-imbalance-in-women.

Law, Sung Ping. "The Regulation of Menstrual Cycle and its Relationship to the Moon." *Acta Obstetricia et Gynecologica Scandinavica* 65, no. 1 (January 1986): 45–48. doi:10.3109/00016348609158228.

Lawrence, Janna. "NSAID Use May Prevent Fertile Women from Ovulating." *The Pharmaceutical Journal* 294, no. 7868/9 (June 22, 2015). doi:10.1211 /PJ.2015.20068779.

Lenton, Elizabeth A., Britt-Marie Landgren, Lynne Sexton, and Rosemary Harper. "Normal Variation in the Length of the Follicular Phase of the Menstrual Cycle: Effect of Chronological Age." BJOG 91, no. 7 (July 1984): 681–684. doi:10.1111/j.1471-0528.1984.tb04830.x.

Marturana, Amy. "12 Nagging Health Issues You Can Blame on Your Hormones." *Self*. August 24, 2016. https://www.self.com/story/12-signs-of-hormonal-imbalance.

Mayo Clinic. "Basal Body Temperature for Natural Family Planning." Last
    modified November 13, 2018. https://www.mayoclinic.org/tests-procedures
    /basal-body-temperature/about/pac-20393026.

Mayo Clinic. "Endometriosis." Last modified March 23, 2019. https://www.mayoclinic
    .org/diseases-conditions/endometriosis/symptoms-causes/syc-20354656?p=1.

Mayo Clinic. "Uterine Polyps." Last modified July 24, 2018. https://www.mayoclinic.org
    /diseases-conditions/uterine-polyps/symptoms-causes/syc-20378709.

O'Connor, Roisin. "Menstruation Study Finds over 5,000 Slang Terms for 'Period.'"
    Independent. March 1, 2016. https://www.independent.co.uk/life-style/health-and
    -families/menstruation-study-finds-over-5000-slang-terms-for-period-a6905021.html.

Planned Parenthood. "How Do I Know If My Menstrual Cycle Is Normal?" Accessed
    July 31, 2019. https://www.plannedparenthood.org/learn/health-and-wellness
    /menstruation/how-do-i-know-if-my-menstrual-cycle-normal.

Prapas, N., A. Karkanaki, I. Prapas, I. Kalogiannidis, I. Katsikis, and D. Panidis. "Genetics
    of Polycystic Ovary Syndrome." *Hippokratia* 13, no. 4 (Oct-Dec 2009): 216–223.

Smoley, Brian A., and Christa M. Robinson. "Natural Family Planning." *American Family
    Physician* 86, no. 10 (November 15, 2012): 924–928.

Tarkan, Laurie. "The Link Between Infertility and Insulin Resistance." *Endocrine Web*.
    Accessed July 31, 2019. https://www.endocrineweb.com/infertility-insulin-resistance
    -5-tips-your-odds-getting-pregnant.

Telfer, Nicole. "Hypothyroidism and the Menstrual Cycle." *Clue*. September 12, 2018.
    https://helloclue.com/articles/cycle-a-z/hypothyroidism-and-the-menstrual-cycle.

"Uterine Fibroids." US Department of Health and Human Services, Accessed
    September 16, 2019. https://www.womenshealth.gov/a-z-topics/uterine-fibroids.

Varney, Helen. *Varney's Midwifery*. Boston: Jones and Bartlett, 1996.

Wechsler, Toni. *Taking Charge of Your Fertility*. 10th ed. New York: William Morrow
    Paperbacks, 2006.

Williams, T., R. Mortata, and S. Porter. "Diagnosis and Treatment of Polycystic Ovarian
    Syndrome." *American Family Physician* 94 (2016):106–13.

Index

A

Adrenal hormones, 100, 108
Anovulatory cycles, 2, 24, 92
Apps, 17

B

Basal body temperature,
    5, 14, 35–36
Basal Body Temperature
    Charts, 38–85
Basal body thermometers, 4
Biphasic temperature
    shifts, 88
Birth control failure
    rates, 13
Breakthrough bleeding, 24

C

Cervical fluid, 7–9
Charting
  Basal Body Temperature
      Charts, 38–85
  cervical fluid key, 28
  chart comparisons, 90–91
  cheat sheet, 92
  how to, 14, 27
  interpreting results,
      32, 88–89
  menstrual flow key, 28
  patterns in, 10
  sample charts, 29–31
Chemical pregnancies, 23, 34
Corpus luteum, 17, 22
Cortisol, 100, 108
Coverlines, 88–89

E

Endometrial lining, 24
Endometriosis, 96–97,
    104–105
Estrogen
  and basal body
      temperature, 5
  and cervical fluid, 7–8
  and ovulation,
      16–17, 21–22

F

Fertility awareness method,
    13. See also Charting
Fevers, 92
Fibroids, 98, 106–107
Follicle stimulating
    hormones (FSH), 16
Follicular phase, 6, 16,
    21, 34, 88, 91

H

Health care providers, 114
Hormone imbalances,
    100, 108–110

I

Insulin, 100, 111. See
    also Polycystic ovary
    syndrome (PCOS)

L

Lifestyle, 100, 110–112
Lunar cycle, 19–20
Luteal phase, 6, 17, 22, 34, 88

Luteal phase defect, 23
Luteinizing hormones
    (LH), 16–17, 22

M

Menstrual cycle
  and cervical fluid, 7–9
  endometriosis and,
      96–97, 104–105
  hormone imbalances
      and, 100, 108–110
  length of, 10
  lifestyle and, 100,
      111–112
  phases of, 6, 19–22, 34
  polycystic ovary
      syndrome (PCOS) and,
      96–97, 100–103
  start of, 14, 16
  uterine growths and,
      98–99, 106–107
Menstruation phase,
    6, 14, 16, 21
Miscarriage, 23, 34
Moon cycle, 19–20

N

NSAIDs, 112

O

Ovulation, 6, 17, 22,
    34, 35, 88–89

P

Periods, 16–17

Polycystic ovary syndrome (PCOS), 96, 100–103

Polyps, 99, 106–107

Progesterone
  and basal body temperature, 5
  production of, 17, 22

S

Spotting, 21, 24, 28, 32, 36, 92

Stress, 111

Sympto-thermal method, 7

T

Thyroid hormones, 100, 109–110

U

Uterine growths, 98–99, 106–107

Uterine lining, 23–24

W

Weight, 111–112

Acknowledgments

I would like to thank my partner, Evin, for all his support and encouragement not only while I was writing this book but also throughout my career and our life together. It's not an easy path we've chosen, but traveling it with you has made my life better than I ever dreamed possible. Thank you to my daughter Winter, an aspiring author whose passion for all things literature inspired me to try my hand at writing, and to my daughter Willa, whose unbridled enthusiasm and bravery have inspired me to be courageous enough to try. Thank you to my mom for always being proud of me and to my friends and midwife family, whose unanimous agreement that I should write this book gave me the push I needed. Thanks to Jen and Tara for welcoming me into their world of writing and helping me find my voice (and the word count feature) and to Sara for finding my good side. And lastly, thank you to my editors and publisher for giving me the opportunity to write this book and share my love of educating and supporting women.

About the Author

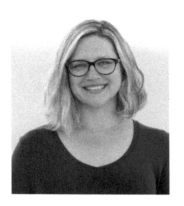

Keeley McNamara, CNM, is a native New Yorker and lifelong vegetarian. She brings a unique mix of New York neurosis and wannabe witchiness to her practice. She works as a midwife in a public hospital, providing care to mostly underserved and undocumented women. What Keeley loves most about midwifery is that it's a perfect mix of activism and medicine. You can find Keeley talking about periods and answering questions most people are too embarrassed to discuss on Instagram @AskMidwifeKeeley.

CPSIA information can be obtained
at www.ICGtesting.com
Printed in the USA
LVHW051030311019
635903LV00002B/4